Human Well-Being Research and Policy Making

Series Editors

Richard J. Estes, School of Social Policy & Practice, University of Pennsylvania, Philadelphia, PA, USA

M. Joseph Sirgy , Department of Marketing, Virginia Polytechnic Institute & State University, Blacksburg, VA, USA

This series includes policy-focused books on the role of the public and private sectors in advancing quality of life and well-being. It creates a dialogue between well-being scholars and public policy makers. Well-being theory, research and practice are essentially interdisciplinary in nature and embrace contributions from all disciplines within the social sciences. With the exception of leading economists, the policy relevant contributions of social scientists are widely scattered and lack the coherence and integration needed to more effectively inform the actions of policy makers. Contributions in the series focus on one more of the following four aspects of well-being and public policy:

- Discussions of the public policy and well-being focused on particular nations and worldwide regions
- Discussions of the public policy and well-being in specialized sectors of policy making such as health, education, work, social welfare, housing, transportation, use of leisure time
- Discussions of public policy and well-being associated with particular population groups such as women, children and youth, the aged, persons with disabilities and vulnerable populations
- Special topics in well-being and public policy such as technology and well-being, terrorism and well-being, infrastructure and well-being.

This series was initiated, in part, through funds provided by the Halloran Philanthropies of West Conshohocken, Pennsylvania, USA. The commitment of the Halloran Philanthropies is to "inspire, innovate and accelerate sustainable social interventions that promote human well-being." The series editors and Springer acknowledge Harry Halloran, Tony Carr and Audrey Selian for their contributions in helping to make the series a reality.

Louise Dalingwater • Vanessa Boullet •
Iside Costantini • Paul Gibbs

Editors

The Unequal Costs of Covid-19 on Well-being in Europe

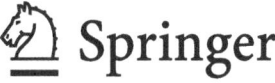

Editors
Louise Dalingwater
Sorbonne Université
Paris, France

Iside Costantini
Department of English Studies
New Sorbonne University
Paris, France

Vanessa Boullet
Department of Foreign Languages and Business
University of Lorraine
Nancy, France

Paul Gibbs
Department of Education
Middlesex University
Hendon, UK

ISSN 2522-5367   ISSN 2522-5375   (electronic)
Human Well-Being Research and Policy Making
ISBN 978-3-031-14424-0   ISBN 978-3-031-14425-7   (eBook)
https://doi.org/10.1007/978-3-031-14425-7

This Springer imprint is published by the registered company Springer Nature Switzerland AG
The registered company address is: Gewerbestrasse 11, 6330 Cham, Switzerland

Acknowledgements

Many thanks to the Springer publishers for their support and guidance. Thank you family and friends.

Contents

List of Figure

List of Tables

Chapter 1
Introduction

Louise Dalingwater, Vanessa Boullet, and Iside Costantini

Countries are still reeling from the effects of the Covid-19 epidemic which has swept across Europe. The current geopolitical situation since the Russian attack on Ukraine has only served to reinforce the crisis. Since March 2020, almost all nations of the world have faced unprecedented changes to their daily lives given the health, economic, and social challenges the pandemic has raised. While the first cases of the novel virus were detected in Wuhan, China, the head of the WHO, Dr. Tedros Adhanom Ghebreyesus, declared Europe to be the epicentre of the global coronavirus pandemic in March 2020, with more cases and deaths reported here at that time than the rest of the world, excluding China (UN, 2020a). The WHO thus urged countries to take decisive and aggressive steps to save lives. Measures taken varied, but they included border closures, restrictions on movement, national lockdowns, closure of schools and universities, curbs on large gatherings, and closure of theatres, restaurant, and bars. Successive waves which have seen similar measures taken in Europe to stem the transmission of the virus have caused further economic and social disruption. Beyond dealing with the human loss of lives, subsequent measures to deal with the crisis can be seen to have a significant impact on mental health and overall well-being.

The notion of well-being itself is very much related to the definition of health as the WHO underlines, that is a "state of complete physical, mental and social

L. Dalingwater (✉)
Sorbonne Université, Paris, France
e-mail: louise.dalingwater@sorbonne-universite.fr

V. Boullet
University of Lorraine, Nancy, France
e-mail: vanessa.boullet@univ-lorraine.fr

I. Costantini
Université Sorbonne Nouvelle, Paris, France
e-mail: iside.costantini@sorbonne-nouvelle.fr

© The Author(s), under exclusive license to Springer Nature Switzerland AG 2022   1
L. Dalingwater et al. (eds.), *The Unequal Costs of Covid-19 on Well-being in Europe*,
Human Well-Being Research and Policy Making,
https://doi.org/10.1007/978-3-031-14425-7_1

well-being and not merely the absence of disease or infirmity" (WHO, 1946). But there is still no commonly agreed definition of well-being. Some consider well-being to be equivalent to happiness (Layard, 2005). Others relate the concept to life satisfaction, quality of life, and sustainability (OECD, 2014; Scott, 2012). Subjective well-being or happiness is said to incorporate three main components: first, life satisfaction which can be gauged by asking people how happy they are overall with their life; second, positive emotions and an absence or low level of negative emotions; third, such notions are also completed by psychological well-being and *eudaimonic* well-being (Diener, 2000; Argyle, 2001).

A wealth of measures to monitor well-being have emerged in the twenty-first century in Europe and beyond. The Eurofound surveys have studied quality of life in Europe since 2003. Following the publication of the Stiglitz report (Stiglitz et al., 2009), the Council of Europe included the concept of well-being for all its members as part of a new strategy for social cohesion, which was approved by the Committee of Ministers. These measures have been used to assess the impact of Covid-19 and measures of containment on people's lives. Eurofound's e-survey, *Living, working and Covid-19*, for example, has sought to provide a snapshot of the impact of the pandemic on people's lives (Eurofound, 2020). It is hoped that providing such information will enable policymakers to bring about an equal recovery from the crisis. The first of these Covid-19 e-surveys was launched on 9 April 2020 while many European countries were still in lockdown, then the second round was conducted in July 2020 when many of the containment measures were relaxed. Since then it has continued to publish reports in the field. The data include life satisfaction, happiness, optimism and resilience, health, support and well-being and trust in institutions across EU countries.

While such attempts to measure the impact of the current health crisis and provide appropriate policy responses are laudable, these new measures of well-being which have emerged over the last two decades essentially place too much emphasis on subjective well-being or "deliberative" utilitarianism. This tends to move our focus away from other more objective concerns linked to inequality or welfare (Gadrey, 2012). Subjective well-being is closer to the sense of economic utility, relating to "personal benefit gained by an individual from a particular interaction or a particular behavior" (Eichhorn, 2013). Since the 1980s, neoliberal policies promoted in many countries across Europe can explain the current context of well-being with a preference for less generous social welfare and a greater need to measure individual well-being (Scott, 2012; Eichhorn, 2013; Coron & Dalingwater, 2017; Dalingwater et al., 2019).

1.1 Economic and Social Structures and Well-Being During the Coronavirus Pandemic

Radcliffe posits that there is a strong positive connection between life satisfaction and welfare. He calls for the strengthening of economic and social structures through state intervention because well-being is enhanced when the state intervenes to reduce market dependence through the decommodification of labour and the adoption of a social democratic welfare regime. According to Esping-Andersen (1990), generous welfare states mean that if individuals have to stop work or decide to opt out of work, it will not have a significant impact on their overall well-being. Pacek and Radcliffe (2008) contend that welfare states contribute to enhancing human well-being.

Economic and social systems in Europe have had to deal with the long-run harm that the current pandemic has inflicted on populations. The significant economic downturn will have a durable effect on health and income even for those who are lucky not to be infected. The burden on healthcare systems, government assistance programmes, and overall welfare is significant. This is because the current health crisis has led to a wide-scale economic crisis. In January 2022, the IMF cut its global growth forecast to 4.4% for 2022. But since then, it has revised previsions following the war in Ukraine. The world economy is experiencing ravaging inflation, financial tightening and the effects of further lockdowns in China which impact on European supply chains. As a result, they have projected a further downgrade for global growth for the rest of 2022 and 2023 (IMF, 2022).

Apart from the economic scars, evidence from the 1918 influenza pandemic has shown that exposure from disease can lead to lifetime health problems either directly related to contamination or the economic effects (lay-offs, etc.) of the disease. The costs are supported not only directly by individuals but households, communities, and even future generations. It is also evident from the analysis of the Great Depression that those entering the labour market in times of great upheaval experience economic penalties long after the crisis has passed. The analysis of historic economic and health crises thus underscores that there is a two-way linkage between the economy and health. Damage to health can undermine performance on the labour market, and economic damage which directly affects labour market prospects can consequently undermine health in the long run. Furthermore, low-income countries and, in particular, marginalized populations will bear the brunt of the current health crisis and economic downturn.

1.2   Structural Inequalities and Well-Being During Covid-19

The complexity of the crisis thus represents both a double economic and health threat to European populations (Grasso et al). While large-scale interventions have come from governments across Europe, the impact of the crisis has been felt unevenly across sectors of society. Societies which have weaker welfare systems tend to be those that have increased inequalities. Prior to the crisis, world leaders recognized that inequality is a cause of social and economic harm (Since the beginning of the sanitary crisis, inequalities have widened in many countries.

The WHO (2020) reports that the uneven impact of Covid-19 had not been fully anticipated or considered in many government response plans. This has put vulnerable populations at a significant risk in the short and medium term, increasing economic and social inequities for the long term. As Gupta et al. (2021) argue, previous flaws in societal governance and the global socio-economic system have meant that we are not just facing a specific health crisis at present but multi-layered crises. While significant policy measures were put in place to protect populations from infection (quarantine, testing, tracing, school and business closures, mass distribution of personal protective equipment and vaccine roll outs) certain populations remain excluded from these measures depending on location and social groups (Ghosal et al., 2020; Gupta et al., 2021).

While lockdowns helped reduce the spread of infection, it also shut down local food systems, disrupted food supplies and led to an increase in prices (Béné, 2020; Farcas et al., 2021). The self-employed and those on temporary, short-term contracts were often significantly affected by the effects of lockdown (Douglas et al., 2020; Gupta et al., 2021). The WHO underlines that Covid-19 and the subsequent containment measures have increased existing inequities in many ways because vulnerable populations are likely to suffer from more serious health impacts because of pre-existing health conditions or because of barriers to accessing health services. The economic and social effects of the crisis can in turn also seriously impact vulnerable populations' overall well-being (WHO, 2020).

While distribution of vaccines has been fairly widespread, significant difficulties remain in terms of ensuring that poor countries but also poorer communities in Europe are able to access vaccines in a timely manner. High-income countries only represent 13% of the population, but they have obtained the lion's share of Covid-19 vaccines (Rutschman, 2021). With high-income countries including those in Europe ensured protection, the fact that there are significant public health inequalities between the global North and global South and within European countries is a cause for concern.

Grasso et al. (2021) argue that significant health impairment, psychological, social, and economic consequences across European societies have had an impact on both material and subjective well-being. They also show evidence that vulnerable communities have been particularly at risk. The effects of the crises have thus deepened inequalities and had an uneven impact on certain categories of populations, namely, women, caregivers, migrants, and other vulnerable persons.

1.2.1 A Widening of Gender Inequalities

Covid-19 has exacerbated a number of pre-existing socio-economic inequalities for women (Ewing-Nelson, 2020). Moreover, women's employment has been more at risk compared to men's in this current pandemic with much greater job losses (Alon et al., 2020; IWPR, 2020). Moreover, since women typically comprise the majority of health and social care workers, they have also been particularly exposed to infection (UN, 2020a). While some of these losses are related to company redundancy plans, some women have also been forced to leave their jobs to respond to higher childcare needs because of school and day care closures. In parallel, women's share of unpaid care work has increased at a significantly higher rate (Alon et al., 2020). Women tend to be more often in part-time jobs with less secure conditions (access to health insurance, sick leave, or other benefits) (Poteat et al., 2020). An increase in unpaid work or a significantly higher burden of both unpaid and paid work can have an impact on psychological well-being (Fortier, 2020). Women have also been found to suffer from greater psychological distress as caregivers than men (Fortier, 2020). Quitting jobs or reducing working time will have an impact on women's well-being (reduced pay, benefits, and opportunities) well beyond the duration of the current pandemic (Fortier, 2020). Previous studies have indeed shown that both men and women have reduced well-being if they are obliged to exit the labour market.

Much of the literature has thus underlined how women's life satisfaction has diminished as a result of more intense domestic and childcare activities, including homeschooling, as a result of lockdown measures. A study carried out by Kulic et al. (2021) of women and unpaid work during the crisis in Germany and Hungary shows how women have increased domestic and childcare duties since the beginning of the crisis. Czymara et al. (2021)'s study noted a significant increase in stress related to extra domestic work for women. Reichelt et al. (2021)'s study shows that women were more vulnerable to labour market dislocation than men. Indeed, they point to a study which included Germany as one of the focus countries and found that women were more likely to reduce their working hours and be made redundant as a result of the pandemic than men. Prior to the pandemic, these women had already been experiencing precarious employment situations. Minello et al. (2021) show that women in academia feared that progress in their careers would be affected because of a decline in research outcomes and publications during a period in which they have had additional domestic and childcare responsibilities. Such inequalities were deeper according to one study depending on the employment and social policies in place across Europe and governmental support provided during the crisis (Cook & Grimshaw, 2020). For example, in Germany parents did not have access to emergency childcare like in France or the UK, which led to increased stress and a greater care burden for women.

1.2.2 The Widening of Workplace Inequalities Faced with Coronavirus

Besides the significant impact on women, those of lower social classes are generally reported to be more at risk from the negative economic and health repercussions in the workplace. Holst et al.'s (2021) study reported that these class inequalities were amplified during the coronavirus crisis. Indeed, the pandemic has different consequences on the ratio risks/occupation and on employment and incomes even in the most developed economies.

Walsh et al.'s (2020) study shows that there were large differences in the risks of having Covid-19 depending on the occupations of the workers. Evidence suggests that the workers at the lower end of the income distribution suffered the most for different reasons (UN, 2020b).

First, labour market protection is minimal for a majority of lower-income workers: many are paid by the hour (on short-term contract), with little or no paid sick leave. With the pandemic, millions of workers saw their working hours reduced, feared for their job, or, even worse, became redundant in the different consumer sectors, which meant a huge loss of income for the household, leading for some of them to poverty. With the pandemic, the demand for labour completely collapsed and, once unemployed, it was almost impossible to find a new job. Moreover, in many European countries, despite the automatic stabilizers of welfare states, the short-time work allowance did not fully compensate for the loss of earnings. According to the UN (2020a), "in hard-hit Italy and Spain, an estimated 27% and 40% of the population, respectively, do not have enough savings to allow themselves not to work for more than 3 months, even if they are only living on the poverty line; and the number is an alarming 39% for the OECD average". Many self-employed also experienced a drop in sales and profits and saw their economic existence threatened and the state support they received did not fully compensate for the usual earnings (Von Carsten et al., 2020).

Second, to prevent the spread of the virus, it was recommended to work from home. But this option was mainly open to people with high salaries and high qualifications. Working remotely had different consequences depending on the living situation: some were more productive because of an increase in workload, better concentration because of a quieter environment at home, no commuter times, but the majority were less productive, usually for parents with small children who lack external childcare options (Von Carsten et al., 2020). However, a large majority of workers, seen as essential by the governments to ensure the running of society and the economy at the onset of the Covid-19 pandemic, were unable to work remotely, estimated to be about 22% in Ireland and the UK (Farquharson et al., 2020;

Redmond & McGuinness, 2020). As these workers are employed in sectors that require close physical proximity to others in the workplace (interactions with customers or colleagues), they faced greater exposure to the virus (Crowley & Justin, 2020). For example, people working in social care (such as care workers and home carers) were identified to be of particular high risk (ONS, 2020) along with house-keepers, public transport drivers, sales assistants, process plant operatives, security guards, and those involved in food production and/or in the logistics sector as they continued to work on the frontline even during lockdowns. The ONS (2020) shows that in England and Wales, over 27% of Covid-19 deaths among those aged 20–64 were employed in these occupations (ONS, 2020; Williams, 2020).

Likewise, gig and sex workers were very vulnerable. Indeed, a study carried out between March and April 2020 in France of precarious workers (Apouey et al., 2020) particularly those working in the gig economy who could not rely on stable incomes and were excluded from employee labour protection, found that these workers had been particularly exposed to wage decreases owing mainly to lock-downs. More than half were reported to have stopped work and a third experienced a fall in wages.

Moreover, as many of those essential workers are older, live in more deprived areas, and have greater rates of chronic illness, the risks of severe outcomes from Covid-19 (e.g. hospitalization and death) are greater (Walsh et al., 2020).

Thus, the association of limited labour market protection and close physical proximity to others means that the low-wage workers, when they were not unem-ployed, were more harmed by the epidemic, in terms of both economic and health outcomes. As the UN said (2020a), "the vicious cycle between low socio-economic status and high health risk could exacerbate the high levels of income inequality in many countries".

1.2.3 Frontline Workers Taking an Uneven Share of the Burden

Other vulnerable persons that have emerged from this pandemic are frontline healthcare professionals. They have seen their workload increase and had to work with inadequate medical resources. They are also one of the most exposed populations to infection. They may also fear infecting people around them and have in some countries also suffered from discrimination. They often suffer from significant stress, anxiety, or depression. While health and social care workers are considered to play a major role in taking care of the sick during Covid-19, previous studies have shown that they already suffer from a high rate of mental health disorders (Gold, 2020; Petrie et al., 2019; Nguyen et al., 2020), which may have a negative impact on patient care. Studies on previous outbreaks have shown that such conditions may worsen during infectious outbreaks (Maunder et al., 2006; Brooks et al., 2018; De Kock et al., 2021).

De Kock et al.'s (2021) systematic review of 24 studies indicated that Covid-19 has had a considerable impact on the psychological well-being of frontline hospital staff. Nurses are shown to be at particularly high risk of adverse mental symptoms resulting from the pandemic. They note that some specific features of the Covid-19 specifically increase the adverse impacts on Health and Social Care Workers, due to both the scale (the vast number of cases to treat) and the number of countries affected. Media have accentuated the focus on deaths and the destructive nature of the pandemic. Work patterns have also been disrupted to a large extent for health and social care workers who have to work outside their usual schedule and workplace (changing departments, for example).

1.2.4   Students' Health Inequalities and Prospects on the Job Market: The Future Workforce Shaken

Those in full-time education have also been significantly affected by the Covid-19 crisis. All G20 countries made the decision to end in-person instruction and move to online communication. Most study abroad programmes were cancelled and international students were asked to return home. International students were basically left with the choice to remain in their host country (sometimes in empty residence halls) or return to their home countries (Nurunnabi et al., 2021).

In Europe, both staff and students had to quickly adapt to a new online environment but many lacked support, skills, and equipment in sufficient quantity (Grasso et al., 2021). Not all schools and universities were well equipped in terms of infrastructure, devices, and human capital to cope with the challenge of offering digital education. According to UNESCO, only 20% of countries were equipped with online teaching devices and programmes before the pandemic. Schooling systems were not digitally prepared, revealing the overall weakness of European digital learning (Irien, 2021). In the European Union, education policies remain the exclusive sphere of national countries which explains why the response to such challenges differed considerably. In Romania, for instance, schools were closed for an average of 32 weeks between 2020 and 2021, but only 6 out of 10 students were provided with online education. In the UK, one in five students was unable to access online learning. Some countries, such as Sweden, seemed to be better equipped as their government had already developed hybrid forms of education prior to the pandemic (Irien, 2021).

Even for those learning institutions which were well equipped at the start, it did not necessarily lead to an appropriate quality education. For instance, an Italy Education expert states that "about 70–75% of teachers did not know how to [teach their students online]. [. . .]. And so, they connected to their students through video calls. But they didn't know the right approach because they thought that it was only a way to move school from class to video calls" (Donoso & Retzmann, 2021). The previously in-person teaching method could not simply be transferred to an online class where the setting is different. This explains why teachers needed support from their institutions. In the UK, the Irish National Digital Experience Survey reveals that 70% of academics were completely inexperienced in online teaching before the crisis even if a majority of teachers felt they had received adequate support from their institutions (Irien, 2021).

At the same time, not all students had sufficient access to equipment or a reliable Internet connection at home. A recent UN policy brief explains how "in most European countries, children from lower socio-economic backgrounds are more likely to lack reading opportunities, a quiet room, and parental support during school closure" (Donoso & Retzmann, 2021). Some universities like Staffordshire in the North West of England have a higher percentage of students facing digital poverty and lack of space which puts a further strain on studies (*The Guardian*, January 2021) and leads to severe inequalities between campuses depending not only on the facilities of the campus but also on the background of enrolled students.

More generally speaking, the pandemic throws a spotlight on other dimensions of inequality. Closing schools also makes the digital divide more pronounced as in the example of Romania. Students who are on the wrong side of the divide are not able to take full advantage of remote learning. The digital divide could translate into an educational divide, with possible long-term consequences (UN, 2020a).

Lockdown, social distancing, and self-isolation requirements are stressful and detrimental for many individuals and have caused students' health and well-being concerns (Grasso et al., 2021). Almost two thirds of students in the UK say their mental health is worse off because of the pandemic according to a national survey undertaken by Hepi (Hewitt, 2021). Students were badly hit in terms of health during the lockdown with reduced movement and opportunities to socialize but the associations which have led to a deterioration of health are yet to be determined (Savage et al., 2000). Female students are at higher risk of facing negative mental effects of the lockdown but only at a smaller effect size (Lischer et al., 2021).

Furthermore, students' health and well-being issues were not necessarily addressed by all G20 countries in a homogeneous fashion. The UK has placed health and well-being in general on its national priority agenda and therefore compares favourably to G20 countries which did not provide any specific policies to address students' health and well-being needs during the pandemic (Nurunnabi et al., 2021). In 2006, Universities UK (UUK)/GuildHE which represent university bodies published a framework for institutional mental health policy for students in higher education to be adopted by all UK universities in the network. The UK has developed an all-inclusive approach since 2016 which recommends that all aspects of university life promote and support student and staff mental health (Nurunnabi et al., 2021, p. 66).

According to the *Journal of Public Health Research* contributors, G20 countries should also integrate international students better in their plan. For instance, the experience of studying in the UK during a pandemic was rated as bad by 61% of Chinese students who took part in the survey and this reaction could affect future generations' choice of destination (*The Pie News*, April 2021). A clear fall in the number of foreign students notably Chinese students who represent the biggest share in the international market (102,000 as of 2019–20, House of Commons Library 2021) could be worrying for the mid-term stability of the UK educational system. Isolation especially for foreign students or migrants' offspring generated further difficulties and the lack of social interaction meant they could not really turn elsewhere for help or a model (Grasso et al., 2021). Indeed, the outcome of the "coping process" mostly relies on personal resources, social and emotional support (Babicka-Wirkus et al., 2021). "To raise the quality and inclusiveness of education and training systems and the provision of digital skills for all", the European Commission launched the new Digital Education Action Plan for the year 2021 to 2027. Through this plan, the Commission's objective is to "learn from the Covid-19 crisis and make education and training systems fit for the digital age". The Covid-19 crisis has had as an effect to push education more to the frontline and accelerate changes within European educational systems to make them more in line with the current digitalization taking place in society and the workplace (European Commission, 2021).

1.2.5   A Widening of Inequalities for Ethnic Minorities

Some studies have focused on the widening of inequalities for ethnic minorities and migrants. The sanitary crisis has worsened the already existing migrant crisis which began in 2015 (Bozorgmehr et al., 2020). The failure to settle asylum seekers across Europe and a lack of solidarity within the EU have led to a struggle to manage migrants from a financial, technical, and institutional perspective, particularly in border countries such as Italy and Greece. Significant SARS Covid-19 outbreaks were reported in overcrowded refugee camps and migrant hostels (Bozorgmehr et al., 2020). Hygiene measures for the vulnerable such as hand washing, restricting social mobility, *etc.*, are extremely difficult for those living in overcrowded accommodation or poor housing conditions with lack of adequate sanitation or easy access to health care services. Migrant workers who are obliged to travel to work were also at risk (day labourers, vulnerable migrants . . .) (Brown et al., 2016; Gupta et al., 2021).

Minority groups and the homeless are particularly vulnerable to new viruses and diseases. It is more difficult to detect cases and prevent the spread of disease in crowded and insalubrious dwellings. In some countries, the infrastructure and resources to shelter these persons were lacking. Overcrowded prisons and detention centres have shown to spread coronavirus. Migrant children were also seen to face particular challenges and experience learning difficulties (Popyk & Pustułka, 2022).

In the UK, ethnic minority communities have been reported to suffer from systemic disadvantages, such as overcrowded living conditions, poor housing, and high exposure to the virus at home and at work (Marmot et al., 2020). In Germany, migrants of Asian, Turkish, or former Yugoslavian backgrounds were found to have great health risks than natives.

Discrimination towards Chinese migrants and their descendants was the subject of a number of studies: one focusing on France (Wang et al., 2021) and another on the UK and Russia (Murji & Picker, 2021). A study carried out by Falkenhain et al. (2021) showed how the crisis had increased uncertainty for refugees in everyday working life. Migrant populations may also be victims of xenophobia and other discrimination. They have even been accused in some cases of spreading the disease.

1.2.6 Regional Health Divisions Exposed Even Further

Risk factors and likelihood of catching the disease also depend on locality. A number of papers have studied the spread of Covid-19 and the economic and socio-demographic determinants of the spread of disease at the local level (Ginsburgh et al., 2021). In the USA, Borjas (2020) reported that those living in poorer and immigrant neighbourhoods and/or those living in large households had a higher chance of becoming affected. Verwimp (2020) in his study of Belgium also confirms that population density, age structure, and poorer populations have an impact on the contamination rates. Sá (2020)'s study of England and Wales reported a positive correlation between Covid-19 mortality and population density age and the presence of minorities (black and Asian populations). Poor housing arrangements in these communities tended to increase the risk of infection. Ginsburgh et al.'s study of French sub-regions shows that inequalities within the sub-regions led to increased exposure and death from Covid-19. In particular, an increase by 1% in the Gini coefficient in a department of France led to a 0.1% increase in death or hospitalization (Ginsburgh et al., 2021).

Some studies have shown that already existing health and social inequalities across regions have widened during Covid-19. For example, the Marmot review (2020), which is a update of the 2010 review of health inequalities in the UK, underscores how health inequalities reported by comparing life expectancies in deprived areas have worsened. Covid-19 mortalities, for example, were higher in those areas which had been already identified as reporting lower life expectancies. There is strong evidence from some countries that those who live in more deprived areas have higher rates of Covid-19 infection rates and mortality. In England and Wales, those living in the most deprived areas have much higher rates of Covid-19 incidence and mortality. Covid-19 mortality rates are 30% higher in the most deprived deciles compared to the least deprived decile (ONS, 2020).

1.3 Focus of the Book

When estimating the costs to well-being as a result of the outbreak of the pandemic and measures implemented to stem transmission, the authors of this volume will thus pay attention to the wider well-being impacts within European countries. In particular, this volume will consider to what extent Covid-19 and measures taken to cope with the crisis have weakened economic and social structures across Europe and what effect this has had on people's lives. While many countries in Europe have reallocated public funding to health care, provided support to SMEs, vulnerable populations and regions hit by the crisis, the well-being or welfare costs (if we take well-being in this broader sense) still risk to be significant. Our assessment will thus go beyond the subjective well-being discourse and evaluate to what extent structural weaknesses within economic, social, and regional frameworks have deepened. It thus recognizes that structural inequalities are key drivers of well-being. This publication contains original contributions which take into account the specific cultural aspects of European and border regions, and how these have come into play to impact on citizens' well-being during Covid-19.

The book is divided into three main parts. The first part explores economic inequalities which have widened since the Covid-19 outbreak. Ted Schrecker's contribution on the United Kingdom in a comparative perspective highlights how the pandemic has resulted in the intensification of both inequalities in economic security and health outcomes. This has come in the form of economically and racially patterned differences in infection, hospitalization, and mortality rates as well as gendered impacts on daily routines and economic futures. Lazarashvili et al.'s chapter shows how, in Georgia, the decline in incomes has had a particularly unequal impact on low-income families, so their socio-economic situation has worsened and they have become even poorer than they were before the pandemic. So, the situation has impacted on the welfare of the country's population and affected the country's tourism, trade, transport, construction, industry, leisure, and entertainment industries and the people employed in them. Turning to the labour market in Germany, Brigitte Lestrade's contribution is much more upbeat noting a limited impact on inequalities in the labour market in this country thanks to reforms predating the Covid crisis. She does however note the uneven burden of informal care for women in this country. Finally, in this part, Boullet and Guillaumond demonstrate how the authorities in Ireland have endeavoured to reduce the unequal consequences of the pandemic on people and economic sectors, while simultaneously trying to improve well-being. However, pre-existing inequalities have meant that the Covid-19 pandemic has hit some segments of the population, particularly the young generation who have experienced reduced job opportunities and increased mental health issues.

The second part is focused on the impact on education and student well-being during Covid-19 and the enduring impact. In Costantini's comparative study of the UK and Hong Kong, after illustrating the major changes which have impacted on student and academics' well-being during Covid-19, namely as a result of the virtualization of higher education, the author suggests that there will most certainly be significant long-term impacts of the Covid-19 pandemic. Remote working and virtual exchanges have given rise to blended learning beyond the initial stages of the pandemic with both positive and negative impacts. However, the unequal impact on the future for certain students resulting from the crisis is unavoidable. Pyzalski and Walter's chapter studies outcomes of the pandemic on young people in Poland who have been particularly sensitive to the effects of Covid-19, namely young people with special needs and their siblings, young people experiencing negative home situations, etc. Despite a number of inevitable difficulties to adapt to online learning, the authors note that some of these vulnerable young people actually experienced numerous positive outcomes which had a positive impact on their functioning and development. A similar study conducted by Verdiyeva et al. in Azerbaijan in the current volume on the impact of the Covid-19 pandemic on the well-being of children with disabilities and their parents notes however that there has been a fundamental uneven impact on children with neurodevelopmental problems. Children with attention deficit/hyperactivity disorder (ADHD), autism spectrum disorder (ASD), and other developmental disabilities proved to be particularly vulnerable to stress due to significant changes in routine and service access and this negatively impacted on their well-being.

The third and final part of this volume looks more specifically at the health inequalities resulting from the Covid-19 epidemic. Lillo-Crespo aims to give a voice to health professionals in Europe to understand their experience of day-to-day practice and to consider how they have coped with the uneven impact of the epidemic on both the population and health care workers. Finally, Dalingwater et al.'s study of the impact of Covid-19 among marginalized migrants in three European countries (France, Sweden, and the UK) shows that migrant well-being has significantly decreased since the outbreak of Covid-19 in Europe and that policy measures to help those marginalized populations have been insufficient. The long-term health effects that such a decline might have in the future are of particular concern.

The collection of articles on specific nations across Europe and on the fringes thus allows us to reflect on significant inequalities during and beyond the Covid-19 pandemic. The chapters also consider how public health mandates may well have adversely affected the plight of vulnerable populations. The chapters also consider a number of lessons which may be learnt from such experiences and how public policy might better develop policies to attempt at counteracting the perceived negative effects on populations in Europe.

References

Alon, T. M., Doepke, M., Olmstead-Rumsey, J., & Tertilt, M. (2020). *The impact of COVID-19 on gender equality*. NBER Working Paper, 26947.

Apouey, B., Roulet, A., Solal, I., et al. (2020). Gig workers during the Covid-19 Crisis in France: Financial precarity and mental well-Being. *Journal of Urban Health, 97*, 776–795. https://doi.org/10.1007/s11524-020-00480-4

Argyle, M. (2001). *The psychology of happiness* (2nd ed.). Routledge. https://doi.org/10.4324/9781315812212

Babicka-Wirkus, A., Wirkus, L., Stasiak, K., & Kozlowski, P. (2021). University students' strategies of coping with stress during the coronavirus pandemic: Data from Poland. *PLoS One Collection*. https://doi.org/10.1371/journal.pone.0255041

Béné, C. (2020). Resilience of local food systems and links to food security – A review of some important concepts in the context of COVID-19 and other shocks. *Food Security, 12*, 1–18. https://doi.org/10.1007/s12571-020-01076-1

Borjas, G. J. (2020). *Demographic determinants of testing incidence and Covid-19 infections in New York city neighborhoods.* NBER Working Paper Series, National Bureau of Economic Research. Working Paper 26952). http://www.nber.org/papers/w26952

Bozorgmehr, K., Saint, V., Kaasch, A., Stuckler, D., & Kentikelenis, A. (2020). Covid and the convergence of three crises in Europe. *The Lancet. Public Health, 5*(5), e247–e248. https://doi.org/10.1016/S2468-2667(20)30078-5

Brooks, S. K., Dunn, R., Amlôt, R., Rubin, G. J., & Greenberg, N. (2018). A systematic, thematic review of social and occupational factors associated with psychological outcomes in healthcare employees during an infectious disease outbreak. *Journal of Occupational and Environmental Medicine, 60*(3), 248–257. https://doi.org/10.1097/JOM.0000000000001235

Brown, C., Ravallion, M., & van de Walle, D. (2016). A poor means test?: Econometric targeting in Africa. *Policy Research Working Paper* no. 7915. World Bank. https://openknowledge.worldbank.org/handle/10986/25814

Cook, R., & Grimshaw, D. (2020). A gendered lens on COVID-19 employment and social policies in Europe. *European Societies, 0*(0), 1–13.

Coron, C., & Dalingwater, L. (2017). *Well-being: Challenging the Anglo-Saxon hegemony.* Presses Sorbonne Nouvelle.

Crowley, F., & Justin, D. (2020). Covid-19, occupational social distancing and remote working potential: An occupation, sector and regional perspective. *Regional Science Policy and Practice, 12*, 1211–1234. https://doi.org/10.1111/rsp3.12347

Czymara, C. S., Langenkamp, A., & Cano, T. (2021). Cause for concerns: Gender inequality in experiencing the COVID-19 lockdown in Germany. *European Societies, 23*(sup1), S68–S81. https://doi.org/10.1080/14616696.2020.1808692

Dalingwater, L., Costantini, I. & Champroux, N. (Ed.) (2019). Well-being: Political discourse and policy in the Anglosphere. *Papers in Political Economy*, Université de Québec à Montréal, 62, June 2019 (special issue).

De Kock, J. H., Latham, H. A., & Leslie, S. J. (2021). A rapid review of the impact of Covid-19 on the mental health of healthcare workers: Implications for supporting psychological well-being. *BMC Public Health, 21*, 104. https://doi.org/10.1186/s12889-020-10070-3

Diener, E. (2000). Subjective well-being: The science of happiness and a proposal for a national index. *American Psychologist, 55*(1), 34–43. https://doi.org/10.1037/0003-066X.55.1.34

Donoso, V., & Retzmann, R. (2021, March 10). *The impact of the COVID-19 crisis: Is online teaching increasing inequality and decreasing well-being for children? Parenting for a Digital Future.* https://blogs.lse.ac.uk/parenting4digitalfuture/2021/03/10/Covid19-and-well-being.

Douglas, M., Katikireddi, S. V., Taulbut, M., McKee, M., & McCartney, G. (2020). Mitigating the wider health effects of covid-19 pandemic response. *British Medical Journal, 369*, m1557. https://doi.org/10.1136/bmj.m1557

Eichhorn, J. (2013). Where happiness varies: Recalling Adam Smith to critically assess the UK government project Measuring National Well-being. *Sociological Research Online, 9*(2). http//:www.socresonline.co.uk/19/2/6/html

Esping-Andersen, G. (1990). *The three worlds of welfare capitalism.* Princeton University Press.

Eurofound. (2020). *Living, working and Covid-19. Covid-19 series.* Publications Office of the European Union.

European Commission. (2021). *Digital Education Action Plan (2021-2027).* https://education.ec.europa.eu/focus-topics/digital-education/digital-education-action-plan

Ewing-Nelson, C. (2020). Four times more women than men dropped out of the labor force in September. Factsheet, 2 October. Washington DC: National Women's Law Center. Available at: https://nwlc.org/resources/four-times-more-women-than-men-dropped-out-of-the-labor-force-in-september/. Accessed 16 December 2020.

Falkenhain, M., Flick, U., Hirseland, A., Naji, S., Seidelsohn, K., & Verlage, T. (2021). Setback in labour market integration due to the Covid-19 crisis? An explorative insight on forced migrants' vulnerability in Germany. *European Societies, 23*(sup1), S448–S463. https://doi.org/10.1080/14616696.2020.1828976

Farcas, A. C., Galanakis, C. M., Socaciu, C., Pop, O. L., Tibulca, D., Paucean, A., et al. (2021). Food security during the pandemic and the importance of the bioeconomy in the new era. *Sustainability, 13*(1), 150. https://doi.org/10.3390/su13010150

Farquharson, C., Rasul, I., & Sibieta, L. (2020). *Key workers: Key facts and questions.* IFS Briefing Note BN 285. https://ifs.org.uk/publications/14763

Fortier, N. (2020). COVID-19, gender inequality, and the responsibility of the state. *International Journal of Wellbeing, 3*(10), 77–93.

Gadrey, J. (2012). Croissance, richesse, bien-être, indicateurs: une vidéo de 8 minutes. *Alternative Economiques.* https://blogs.alternatives-economiques.fr/gadrey/2012/10/21/croissance-richesse-bien-etre-indicateurs-une-video-de-8-minutes

Ghosal, S., Bhattacharyya, R., & Majumder, M. (2020). Impact of complete lockdown on total infection and death rates: A hierarchical cluster analysis. *Diabetes & Metabolic Syndrome: Clinical Research & Reviews, 14*(4), 707–711. https://doi.org/10.1016/j.dsx.2020.05.026

Ginsburgh, V., Magerman, G., & Natali, I. (2021). Covid-19 and the role of inequality in French regional departments. *The European Journal of Health Economics, 22,* 311–327. https://doi.org/10.1007/s10198-020-01254-0

Gold, J. A. (2020). Covid-19: Adverse mental health outcomes for healthcare workers. *BMJ, 369,* m1815. https://doi.org/10.1136/bmj.m1815

Grasso, M., Klicperová-Baker, M., Koos, S., Kosyakova, Y., Petrillo, A., & Vlase, I. (2021). The impact of the coronavirus crisis on European societies. What have we learnt and where do we go from here? – Introduction to the Covid volume. *European Societies, 23*(sup1), S2–S32. https://doi.org/10.1080/14616696.2020.1869283

Gupta, J., Bavinck, M., Ros-Tonen, M., Asubonteng, K., Bosch, H., van Ewijk, E., Hordijk, M., Van Leynseele, Y., Lopes Cardozo, M., Miedema, E., Pouw, N., Rammelt, C., Scholtens, J., Vegelin, C., & Verrest, H. (2021). Covid-19, poverty and inclusive development. *World Development, 145,* 105527. https://doi.org/10.1016/j.worlddev.2021.105527

Hewitt, R. (2021, April). *Students' views on the impact of Coronavirus on their Higher Education Experience in 2021.* Higher Education Policy Institute (HEPI). Hepi Policy Note 29. https://www.hepi.ac.uk/wp-content/uploads/2021/03/HEPI-Policy-Note-29-Students-views-on-the-impact-of-Coronavirus-on-their-higher-education-experience-in-2021-26_03_21_pdf

Holst, H., Fessler, A., & Niehoff, S. (2021). Covid-19, social class and work experience in Germany: Inequalities in work-related health and economic risks. *European Societies, 23*(sup1), S495–S512. https://doi.org/10.1080/14616696.2020.1828979

IMF. (2022, April 14). *Facing crisis upon crisis: How the world can respond.* https://www.imf.org/en/News/Articles/2022/04/14/sp041422-curtain-raiser-sm2022

Irien, L. (2021, June 22). Online education in times of Covid-19 – A challenging transition for European countries. *Eyes on Europe* https://www.eyes-on-europe.eu/online-education-in-times-of-Covid-19-a-challenging-transition-for-european-countries/

IWPR (Institute for Women's Policy Research). (2020). *Women are falling further behind men in the recovery and are 5.8 million jobs below pre-COVID employment levels, compared with 5.0 million fewer jobs for men.* Institute for Women's Policy Research. https://iwpr.org/wp-content/uploads/2020/10/QF-Jobs-Day-October-dft-HM-Fact-Checked.pdf [Google Scholar].

Kulic, N., Dotti Sani, G. M., Strauss, S., & Bellani, L. (2021). Economic disturbances in the COVID-19 crisis and their gendered impact on unpaid activities in Germany and Italy. *European Societies, 23*(sup1), S400–S416. https://doi.org/10.1080/14616696.2020.1828974

Layard, R. (2005). *Happiness: Lessons from a New Science.* Penguin Books.

Lischer, S., Netkey, S., & Dickson, C. (2021). Remote learning and students' mental health during the Covid-19 pandemic: A mixed-method enquiry. *Prospects.* https://doi.org/10.1007/s11125-020-09530-w

Marmot, M., Allen, J., Boyce, T., Goldblatt, P., & Morrison, J. (2020). *Health equity in England: The marmot review 10 years on.* Institute of Health Equity.

Maunder, R., Lancee, W., Balderson, K., Bennett, J., Borgundvaag, B., & Evans, S. (2006). Long-term psychological and occupational effects of providing hospital healthcare during SARS outbreak. *Emerging Infectious Diseases, 12*(12), 1924–1932. https://doi.org/10.3201/eid1212.060584

Minello, A., Martucci, S., & Manzo, L. K. C. (2021). The pandemic and the academic mothers: Present hardships and future perspectives. *European Societies, 23*(sup1), S82–S94. https://doi.org/10.1080/14616696.2020.1809690

Murji, K., & Picker, G. (2021). Racist morbidities: A conjunctural analysis of the Covid-19 pandemic. *European Societies, 23*(sup1), S307–S320. https://doi.org/10.1080/14616696.2020.1825767

Nguyen, L. H., Drew, D. A., Graham, M. S., Joshi, A. D., Guo, C., & Ma, W. (2020). Risk of Covid-19 among front-line health-care workers and the general community: A prospective cohort study. *The Lancet: Public Health, 5*(9), e475–e483. https://doi.org/10.1016/S2468-2667(20)30164-X

Nurunnabi, M., Almusharraf, N., & Aldeghaither, D. (2021, Jan 27). Mental health and well-being during the Covid-19 pandemic in higher education: Evidence from G20 countries. *Journal of Public Health Research, 9*(sup1), 2010. https://doi.org/10.4081/jphr.2020.2010

OECD. (2014). *How's life in your region?* OECD.

Office for National Statistics (ONS). (2020). *Coronavirus (Covid-19) related deaths by occupation, England and Wales: Deaths registered up to and including 20 April 2020.* https://www.ons.gov.uk/releases/Covid19relateddeathsbyoccupationenglandandwalesdeathsregistereduptoandincluding20thapril2020

Pacek, A., & Radcliffe, B. (2008). Assessing the welfare state: The politics of happiness. *Perspectives on Politics, 6*(2), 267–277. https://doi.org/10.1017/S1537592708080602

Petrie, K., Crawford, J., Baker, S., Dean, K., Robinson, J., & Venes, B. J. (2019). Interventions to reduce symptoms of common mental disorders and suicidal ideation in physicians: A systematic review and meta-analysis. *The Lancet: Psychiatry, 6*(3), 225–234. https://doi.org/10.1016/S2215-0366(18)30509-1

Popyk, A., & Pustułka, P. (2022). Educational disadvantages during Covid-19 pandemic faced by migrant school children in Poland. *Journal of International Migration and Integration.* https://doi.org/10.1007/s12134-022-00953-2

Poteat, T., Millett, G. A., Nelson, L. E., & Beyrer, C. (2020). Understanding COVID-19 risks and vulnerabilities among black communities in America: The lethal force of syndemics. *Annals of Epidemiology, 47,* 1–3. https://doi.org/10.1016/j.annepidem.2020.05.004

Redmond, P. & McGuinness, S. (2020). *Who can work from home in Ireland? ESRI Survey and Statistical Report Series, 87.* https://www.esri.ie/system/files/publications/SUSTAT87.pdf

Reichelt, M., Makovi, K., & Sargsyan, A. (2021). The impact of COVID-19 on gender inequality in the labor market and gender-role attitudes. *European Societies, 23*(sup1), S228–S245. https://doi.org/10.1080/14616696.2020.1823010

Rutschman, A. (2021). Rutschman Is there a cure for vaccine nationalism? *Current History, 120*(822), 9–14. https://doi.org/10.1525/curh.2021.120.822.9

Sá, F. (2020, May). *Socioeconomic determinants of Covid-19 infections and mortality: Evidence from England and Wales.* CEPR Discussion Paper No. DP14781.

Savage, M. J., Magistro, R., Donaldson, D., Nevill, L. C., Healy, M., & Hennis, P. J. (2000). Mental health and movement behaviour during the Covid-19 pandemic in UK university students: Prospective cohort study. *Mental Health and Physical Activity, 19,* 100357. https://doi.org/10.1016/j.mhpa.2020.100357

Scott, K. (2012). *Measuring well-being: Towards sustainability?* Routledge.

Stiglitz, J., Sen, A. & Fitoussi, J. P. (2009). *Rapport de la commission sur la mesure des performances économiques et du progrès social.* http://www.stiglitz-sen-fitoussi.fr

UN. (2020a, March 13). *Europe is now the new epicenter of the pandemic, according to the WTO.* https://news.un.org/fr/story/2020/03/1063991

UN. (2020b, April). *Covid-19: Disrupting lives, economies and societies.* World Economic Situation and Prospects: Briefing, No. 136. https://www.un.org/development/desa/dpad/publication/world-economic-situation-and-prospects-april-2020-briefing-no-136/

Verwimp, P. (2020). *The Spread of Covid-19 in Belgium: A municipality-level analysis.* Working Papers ECARES 2020-25, ULB (Université Libre de Bruxelles).

Von Carsten, S., Entringer, T., Göbel, J., Grabka, M., Graeber, D., Kröger, H., Kroh, M., Kühne, S., Liebig, S., Schupp, J., Seebauer J. & Zinn, S. (2020, May 12). *Vor dem Covid-19-Virus sind nicht alle Erwerbstätigen gleich.* DIW Berlin. https://www.diw.de/de/diw_01.c.789505.de/publikationen/diw_aktuell/2020_0041/vor_dem_Covid-19-virus_sind_nicht_alle_erwerbstaetigen_gleich.html

Walsh, B., Redmond, P. & Roantre, B. (2020, July). *Differences in risk of severe outcomes from Covid-19 across occupations in Ireland.* ERSI Survey, 93. https://doi.org/10.26504/sustat93.pdf

Wang, S., Chen, X., Li, Y., Luu, C., Ran, Y., & Madrisotti, F. (2021). 'I'm more afraid of racism than of the virus!': Racism awareness and resistance among Chinese migrants and their descendants in France during the Covid-19 pandemic. *European Societies, 23*(sup1), S721–S742. https://doi.org/10.1080/14616696.2020.1836384

WHO. (1946). *Preamble to the Constitution of the World Health Organization as adopted by the International Health Conference.* New York, 19–22 June, 1946; signed on 22 July 1946 by the representatives of 61 States. Official Records of the World Health Organization, no. 2, p. 100) and entered into force on 7 April 1948.

World Health Organization Regional Office for the Eastern Mediterranean (WHO EMRO). (2020). *Zoonotic disease: Emerging public health threats in the Region.* Retrieved May 25, 2020, from http://www.emro.who.int/about-who/rc61/zoonotic-diseases.html

Williams, M. (2020, May 19). Coronavirus class divide – the jobs most at risk of contracting and dying from COVID-19. *The Conversation.* https://theconversation.com/coronavirus-class-divide-the-jobs-most-at-risk-of-contracting-and-dying-from-covid-19-138857

Louise Dalingwater is a full professor of British politics at Sorbonne Université. Her current research focuses on health policy, healthcare delivery and well-being in the United Kingdom, with some comparative research on European health systems (notably France) and global health policy research. Recent publications include a book on the UK service economy, a monograph on the NHS, and several book chapters and articles on well-being and health. She has coedited two publications on well-being: *Well-being: Challenging the Anglo-Saxon Hegemony* (Presses Sorbonne Nouvelle, 2017) and *Well-being: Political Discourse and Policy in the Anglosphere* (Papers in Political Economy, 2019). She is part of the Precision Health Network (an international research project led by the Universities of Lund and Malmo in Sweden). She is also Chair of the Health Wellness and Society Research Network based in Illinois, United States.

Vanessa Boullet is an associate professor at the University of Lorraine. Her research focuses on Irish studies and on the interactions between economy, society, and politics. Her thesis entitled "Planning in Ireland (1958–1972), methodologies and mythology of economic modernisation" was awarded the Prix Richelieu by the Chancellerie des Universités de Paris in 2009. She has developed an interest in the impact of multinationals on the Irish economy and its uneven development. She also tries to develop research in Business and Foreign Languages departments in France and she is a member of the editorial board of the journal *Revue International des Langues Appliquées Etrangères.*

Iside Costantini is an associate professor in British Politics/Civilization at the Sorbonne Nouvelle University, Paris. She completed a Ph.D. in 2009 on nineteenth century exchanges between Great

Britain and South China (Hong Kong, Canton, Shanghai) through the English-language press. She has developed an interest for Sino-British relations from the nineteenth to the twenty-first centuries including comparative approaches in well-being policies/issues. She contributed a chapter "Confucianism Promoted as an Alternative to the Anglo-Saxon Social-Cultural Model" in *Well-being— Challenging the Anglo-Saxon Hegemony* (Presses Sorbonne Nouvelle, 2017) and coedited an online volume *Well-being: Political Discourse and Policy in the Anglosphere* (Papers in Political Economy, 2019).

Part I
The Economic Impact of Covid-19

Chapter 2
Building Back Worse? The Prognosis for Health Equity in the Post-pandemic World

Ted Schrecker

Abstract The concept of health equity—in a simplified view, socially patterned inequalities in health outcomes that are unfair or unjust and avoidable—originated in the work for the World Health Organization's European regional office, and was foregrounded by the work of WHO's Commission on Social Determinants of Health (2005–2008). Yet as political scientist Julia Lynch observed pre-pandemic, 'systematic efforts to reduce inequalities in the "fundamental causes" of health have been vanishingly rare'. The pandemic brought into vivid focus both inequalities in economic security and vulnerability and inequalities in health outcomes, in the form of economically and racially patterned differences in infection, hospitalization, and mortality rates as well as gendered impacts on daily routines and economic futures.

It might be supposed that an overdue increase in policy attention to reducing those inequalities will characterize the post-pandemic world. More likely, however, is the opposite outcome: a decline in the political salience of health (in)equity and, in most countries, its eventual disappearance from the policy agenda. Adopting the conceptual lens of political economy and drawing primarily from the experience of the United Kingdom, but drawing from other (mainly European) jurisdictions as appropriate, I identify at least four reasons for this prognosis:

1. Increased concentration of wealth at the very top of the economic distribution, in a context where ultra-wealth was already becoming ungovernable and its overt and covert influence on politics outsized. Relatedly,
2. The tendency of the income support and fiscal stimulus programmes implemented in response to the economic contractions associated with lockdowns to inflate asset prices, and therefore the incomes and wealth of asset owners, as observed notably in property and share prices.

T. Schrecker (✉)
Newcastle University, Newcastle upon Tyne, UK

Richard M. Fairbanks School of Public Health, Indiana University, Indianapolis, USA
e-mail: theodore.schrecker@ncl.ac.uk

© The Author(s), under exclusive license to Springer Nature Switzerland AG 2022
L. Dalingwater et al. (eds.), *The Unequal Costs of Covid-19 on Well-being in Europe*,
Human Well-Being Research and Policy Making,
https://doi.org/10.1007/978-3-031-14425-7_2

3. In a less conspicuous process, the upward redistribution of resources from the tax base as a whole (which is ultimately responsible for repayment of pandemic-era borrowing) to the buyers of government bonds—disproportionately, wealthy individuals and large individual investors such as pension funds. Only a strongly progressive tax system could avoid this impact, and they are few and far between.
4. A widespread decline in the ability of democratic institutions to provide the accountability that might ensure renewed interest in health (in)equity.

On the basis of currently available data, probably only the first of these patterns is universal; exceptions may be found to the others. However, it remains to be seen whether the exceptions will be sufficiently influential to ensure that health (in)equity remains on, or returns to, the policy agenda. I conclude with a sketch of the generic policies that would be needed to change the situation identified by Lynch in the post-pandemic world, and leave the reader to judge their (im)probability.

2.1   Introduction: Setting the Stage

Later, as he sat on his balcony eating the dog, Dr Robert Laing reflected on the unusual events that had taken place within this huge apartment building during the previous three months. Now that everything had returned to normal, he was surprised that there had been no obvious beginning, no point beyond which their lives had moved into a clearly more sinister dimension.

The epigraph is the opening of J.G. Ballard's (1975, p. 7) magnificent dystopian novel *High-Rise*, about social skirmishes that became murderous class conflicts within the affluent yet vertically stratified world of a 40-floor tower block. Only as we follow the narrative do we learn that the return to "normal" involves a nightmare world in which bands of surviving residents—and many did not survive—have barricaded themselves into enclaves within an internally demolished structure; all essential services have collapsed; and access to basic requisites of life involves such recourses as cooking and eating the pets of residents whose strategies were less successful. The overall message of this chapter is that *High-Rise* is likely to be a more trustworthy thematic guide to what looks normal in the post-pandemic world than much of the proliferating academic literature on the topic, some of which is cited in what follows. Although the focus of the book is on Europe, my analysis often draws primarily on data from the United Kingdom (UK) and the United States (US)—probably the two large, rich countries that have travelled farthest down the neoliberal economic and social policy road. They were the focus of previous research (Schrecker & Bambra, 2015) using a conceptual repertoire ("neoliberal epidemics") that has since been deployed in subsequent work (Schrecker, 2021).

The repertoire connects macro-scale currents in global political economy with their manifestations within national borders and the consequences for health inequalities: the political economy of health (Birn et al., 2017, Chap. 7). The approach taken here goes further, to consider how those connections affect the political plausibility of measures that would reduce post-pandemic health inequalities, especially by way of acting by way of their "upstream" social determinants (Commission on Social Determinants of Health, 2008; Kelly & Doohan, 2012). The arguments, hypotheses, and conjectures presented here invite further, more systematic comparative work. It is especially important for continental European readers to reject the comforting hypothesis that the excesses observed in the US and the UK "can't happen here"; they could. Neglected here are the broader issues exemplified by the inexcusable failure of rich countries and the institutions they dominate to accelerate vaccine supplies and programming in low- and middle-income countries (Bollyky et al., 2022), although from a global health equity perspective these remain critically important.

Well researched examinations of particular governments' early responses to the pandemic, informed by the usual metrics of comparative politics, are already available (e.g. Greer et al., 2021; Alexander et al., 2021; Baldwin, 2021; Or et al., 2021; Vampa, 2021; Wallenburg et al., 2021). As worthwhile as they are, their longer-term value for understanding the post-pandemic future is likely to be limited, for several reasons. The most basic is the inevitable time lag between acceptance and academic publication. Further, at this writing (May 2022) just over 2 years have elapsed since the start of the pandemic. Overall excess deaths—relative to what would be expected based on patterns from the recent past—are a far more useful indicator of pandemic impacts than are official figures on mortality from Covid-19 infection, as are declines in life expectancy for those jurisdictions with adequate data on this point. Assessments of overall excess deaths, by the *Economist*'s Intelligence Unit and the Institute for Health Metrics and Evaluation (IHME), already suggest that the death toll associated with the pandemic is roughly three times the total of official counts of deaths attributable directly to Covid-19. The IHME researchers estimated that 18.2 million excess deaths occurred worldwide during 2020 and 2021 (Covid-19 Excess Mortality Collaborators, 2022). As of March 21, 2022, the *Economist*'s best estimate of 20.1 million overall excess deaths since the start of the pandemic was more than three times the official global figure of 6.1 million deaths from Covid-19 infection (The Pandemic's True Death Toll, 2022), with wide confidence intervals for many countries because of poor data quality. These differences arise partly because of national differences in recording whether a death was specifically attributable to Covid-19, but more significantly because of the effect of pandemic-driven disruptions of health systems on availability of diagnosis and treatment for other illnesses. Such figures also fail to tell the story of the pandemic and inequality.

2.2 The Pandemic's Unequal Impacts

Socio-economic gradients in health, describing a pattern in which the less privileged or advantaged members of a society suffer from worse health and fewer opportunities to lead healthy lives, are nearly ubiquitous worldwide. In an important analysis based on data through 2020, but since confirmed by abundant additional evidence, Bambra et al. (2021) show that the distribution of health outcomes during the pandemic as a result of differential exposures, susceptibilities, and vulnerabilities conformed to this pattern for at least four reasons. First, inequalities in working conditions meant populations such as low-paid, frontline service workers who were obviously unable to work from home were and are more likely to be infected; they also were often reliant on public transport, associated with another set of exposures because of the unavoidable close proximity of fellow passengers. Many such workers whose jobs were not considered "essential" were disproportionately vulnerable to the economic effects of lockdown-related job loss, and often to economic losses associated with illness given a dramatic variation across the high-income world in entitlement to sickness pay (OECD, 2020b, p. 9). Second, "immune systems weakened by long-term exposures to adverse living and environmental conditions" made people both more susceptible to infection and vulnerable to severe illness. The chronic stresses associated with multiple subaltern status, and the associated "weathering" among such populations as African-Americans, especially those who are older, poor and/or female, are a case in point (Geronimus et al., 2006; Garcia et al., 2021). Third, pre-existing conditions and comorbidities such as diabetes and obesity, which themselves exhibit a socio-economic gradient, made people more vulnerable to severe illness once infected. Fourth, increased transmission was associated with such socially patterned variables as crowded or multigenerational housing, which rendered social distancing impossible while often magnifying work-related exposures and vulnerabilities. The disproportionate death toll among care home residents, especially during the first year of the pandemic (Comas-Herrera et al., 2021),[1] must also be noted as reflecting the implied disposability of that population in many countries.

This simplified rendering of a carefully crafted and documented argument suffices to suggest why (for instance) the death rate from Covid-19 in the UK was more than twice as high in England's most deprived small areas than in the least deprived during the first year of the pandemic (Office for National Statistics, 2021b); why Covid-19 mortality in England and Wales among working-age men in frontline service and "elementary" occupations in 2020 was more than three times as among managers and professionals (Office for National Statistics, 2021a); and why the UK's Black, Asian, and minority ethnic (BAME) communities were disproportionately vulnerable both to Covid-19 infection and to Covid-19 mortality (Cheshmehzangi, 2022).[2] This is a short-term picture, and many of the pandemic's effects on health outcomes and health inequalities, such as those operating by way of health system priorities, have not yet had time to appear. It is hard to overstate the

---

[1] For example, deaths among care home residents accounted for 44% of all Covid-19 deaths during the first year of the pandemic in Austria, 57% in Belgium, 39% in Denmark, 43% in France, 47% in Sweden, and 34% in the UK. The cited source warns against direct comparisons among countries, because of differences in how data were collected.

[2] Similar, sometimes even more dramatic patterns were observed in North America. On the Canadian city of Montréal, where the maps of low household income and high proportion of residents self-identifying as Black are very similar, see Rocha et al. (2020); on the Washington, DC region of the US, see Tan et al. (2022).

importance of this point. In the UK, the number of people on public National Health Service (NHS) waiting lists rose by roughly 50% after the start of the pandemic, extrapolating a long austerity-related trajectory (Dorling, 2022; Walker, 2022), and the senior health minister conceded that the situation would get worse before it got better. A minority of the population with private health insurance, or the ability to pay directly for services—both of which are allowed in the UK—were able at least partly to bypass this obstacle. This situation is likely to repeat in jurisdictions with existing two-tier, public-private health financing structures, and a similar pattern of delayed diagnosis and treatment appears to apply to health systems in multiple countries across the global income spectrum (Arsenault et al., 2022). The effects of these delays on health outcomes and their distribution will take at least a few more years to become evident.

Changes in health inequalities that are driven by social determinants of health (Commission on Social Determinants of Health, 2008; Kelly & Doohan, 2012) may take even longer to materialize. These operate most directly by way of material deprivation: the simple lack of resources necessary to sustain a healthy life, even in some of the world's richest countries. For example, before the pandemic a detailed examination of the cost of healthy diets concluded that they would be unaffordable to many low-income households in 24 European cities (Penne & Goedemé, 2021); food insecurity was increasing throughout the UK (Pool & Dooris, 2021). In a gendered and more nuanced frame, consider how domestic divisions of labour under lockdown affected male and female life trajectories differently, influencing not only occupational prospects but also the crucial variable of economic and logistical ability to leave abusive relationships (Take Your Child to Work (Every) Day, 2021). The body of research evidence is already extensive enough to enable two systematic reviews to conclude that the pandemic has resulted in an increase in domestic violence against women in multiple settings (Kourti et al., 2021; Piquero et al., 2021). Over a longer time frame, pandemic-related magnifications of inequality may operate across generations. For example, the shift to online learning during the pandemic widened educational inequalities (The Pandemic Is Widening, 2020). How will differences in the ability of differently situated households to support children's online learning, related both to divisions of labour within the household and access to such resources as computers, affordable Internet access, and suitable spaces for home study during school shutdowns affect future academic achievement, examination results (which are decisive in jurisdictions like the UK), and subsequent socio-economic trajectories? Thus, long-term comparative assessment of national or sub-national success in pandemic response, even using metrics like excess overall deaths, is seriously premature.

The preceding discussion must be considered against a background of the changing, unpredictable consequences of the Russian invasion of Ukraine and the cost-of-living crisis that it has exacerbated, and provides background for the two central arguments of the chapter. First, even if a resurgence of infections related to premature removal of public health restrictions or involving a new variant from outside the highly vaccinated countries can be avoided—and the latter prospect[3] is taken seriously by prominent global health researchers (Nguyen & Kickbusch, 2021)—the pandemic and policy responses to it will almost certainly worsen the social and economic inequalities that are the primary drivers of health inequalities. The economic dimension is likely to be especially significant. Second, on the best available evidence, and in combination with broader currents in the political environment, most initiatives to reduce health inequalities in the post-pandemic world are probably doomed to failure, especially when viewed in combination with the equally urgent imperative of limiting climate change. The rhetoric of "building back better" post-pandemic that has been promoted by the Organisation for Economic Co-operation and Development (OECD, 2020a) and many other actors,[4] even when well intentioned, is likely to remain just rhetoric, in much the same way that early predictions of radical global economic reform after the financial crisis of 2007–08 rapidly gave way to business as usual.

2.3   The Post-pandemic World and the "Inequality Machine"

In the aftermath of that financial crisis, the editor of *Le Monde Diplomatique* described neoliberal globalization as "[t]he inequality machine [that] is reshaping the planet" (Halimi, 2013). Indeed, financial crises associated with the growing importance of finance as an independent centre of profit (financialization, which was a key dimension of post-1980 globalization; see among many other sources Epstein, 2005; Freeman, 2010; Krippner, 2011) have tended to ratchet up inequality in several ways (UNCTAD, 2017, pp. 93–117). "Even when income inequality does not worsen, the lowest income earners bear the brunt of painful market adjustments and economic policies adopted in response to financial crises" (*Ibid*, p. 104). These tendencies were clearly evident in the wake of the 2007–2008 crisis. Worldwide in 2011, almost 27 million more people worldwide were still unemployed than in 2007, and "one in three workers in the labour force [was] either unemployed or poor", as

---

[3]Considerably more likely in the wake of the refusal by a scientifically illiterate US Congress, in April 2022, to appropriate funds for continuing the United States Agency for International Development (USAID) programme of supporting vaccine delivery in low-income countries (Diamond & Roubein, 2022).

[4]I have not provided an inventory of the features of these proposals, most of which are for now largely speculative. The OECD version is notably short on specifics. For a comparison between two more specific "Green New Deal" proposals and a more radical alternative organized around the contentious idea of degrowth, see Mastini et al. (2021). Just before the pandemic hit, the European Commission (2019) unveiled a proposal for a "European Green Deal" organized around the goal of decarbonizing energy systems by 2050. Another important pre-pandemic, more explicitly equity-oriented set of proposals is presented in UNCTAD (2019). Interestingly, none of these proposals incorporates a specific focus on health inequalities, perhaps suggesting the limited salience of the issue for non-specialist audiences.

defined by a poverty line of US$2/day (International Labour Organization, 2012, p. 31). And by 2019, "whereas it took only one year for the global unemployment rate to jump from 5.0% in 2008 to 5.6% in 2009, the recovery to the levels that prevailed before the global financial crisis [had] taken a full nine years" (International Labour Organization, 2019, p. 2). Meanwhile, the number of "high net worth individuals" (with financial assets worth more than US$1 million) across Europe had recovered to its 2007 (pre-crisis) level of 3.1 million by 2010, and had risen to 5.2 million by 2019 (Capgemini & Merrill Lynch, 2011; Capgemini Research Institute, 2020). That was the situation when the pandemic arrived.

Another important element of the pre-pandemic context was a burgeoning housing affordability crisis (Wetzstein, 2017), consequent to the worldwide financialization of housing (Rolnik, 2020; Blakeley, 2021) as housing became "just another asset class" (van Loon & Aalbers, 2017). Immediate health impacts were associated with "double precarity" of housing and employment (Bentley et al., 2019). The crisis was proximally driven by price increases that were extraordinary in historical perspective (Prime cuts, 2019; European Commission, 2022), but distally by the entry of major national and global corporate investors into housing markets (Rolnik, 2020). As the effects of expansionary fiscal policies that were intended to counteract the destructive consequences of lockdowns combined with low or negative interest rates, many countries saw a continued increase in both purchase prices and rents throughout the pandemic (see, e.g., IMF Blog, 2021; Flynn, 2022). Across the European Union, house prices rose 10% between the fourth quarter of 2020 and the fourth quarter of 2021, with considerably higher increases in some countries— 13.9% in Ireland, 12.2% in Germany, and 18.7% in the Netherlands, for instance (European Commission, 2022). In the UK, average sale prices increased by 18.5% between the end of 2019 and the end of 2021 (Office for National Statistics, 2022), obviously with considerable regional variation,[5] at a time when the effects of Thatcher-era planned shrinkage of the social housing sector through the infamous right-to-buy scheme were still being felt. As this pattern occurred alongside rising private sector rents, one researcher warned in 2021 that "the UK [was] sleepwalking into a potential evictions crisis" (Blakeley, 2021, p. 79). As important as the direct and indirect health effects of precarious housing may be, and these are likely to manifest in many places with growing severity over time, a more far-reaching consequence—indeed, potentially the single most important political impact of the pandemic—involves the effect on political allegiances of inequalities in wealth as between homeowners and the rest of the population. One team of researchers (Adkins et al., 2021, p. 3) had already concluded based on pre-pandemic trends that "sustained inflation of property values . . . has fundamentally shifted the social class structure, from a logic that was structured around employment towards one that is organized around participation in asset ownership and appreciation".

---

[5] In North America, increases were even more extreme, with house prices in the US rising by 33% in the two years after the start of the pandemic, with much higher increases in some regions (Where the Lawns, 2022).

In his magisterial *The Great Leveler*, historian Walter Scheidel (2017) identifies plagues as one of the four categories of violent shocks that have led to reductions in inequality over the *longue durée*. Over the short term, pandemic-related fiscal stimulus and direct income transfer policies actually reduced material deprivation in some jurisdictions (Brewer & Tasseva, 2020; Measuring Poverty, 2021). At the household level, this effect largely vanished with the phasing out of the measures in question (see, e.g., Child Allowance, 2022) and, where they were in effect, the end of eviction moratoria. Although tightening labour markets may prolong the beneficial impacts by way of raising wages (The Battle of the Markups, 2022), these effects are likely to be temporary and cancelled out by such factors as housing precarity. The problem is not just housing costs and tenure, but rather economy-wide inflation and associated cost-of-living crises, driven in the first instance by pandemic-related fiscal stimuli and supply chain disruptions, leading an official watchdog agency in the UK to anticipate "the biggest single financial-year fall in living standards since records began 66 years ago" (Hughes, 2022, p. 6). At this writing, the cost-of-living crisis is worsening the accumulated consequences of rising economic marginalization driven by combinations of changed employment options and, often, a decade of austerity. Considerable international variation exists in both the extent of precarious employment and the related, more general indicator of the prevalence of low-paid work (Thelen, 2019), which varies widely among countries. Before the pandemic, the number of workers in the UK on so-called zero-hours contracts, which guarantee no minimum amount of work in a given week, grew from 168,000 in 2010 to 974,000 at the end of 2019 (Office for National Statistics, 2021c). Simultaneously, a decade of austerity-driven tax and spending reforms in the UK had the effect of shifting resources upward in the income distribution, and disproportionately bleeding resources from poorer regions (Schrecker, 2021), whilst worsening food insecurity (Jenkins et al., 2021) among other adverse outcomes.

The knock-on effects of the war in Ukraine have magnified such impacts. At this writing, the war has had especially serious and immediate effects on energy prices. Fuel poverty threatens many European households, which even before the invasion were facing increases of more than 50% in their energy bills in 2022 because of high demand driven by a post-pandemic economic rebound (What Is Behind Rocketing Natural-Gas Prices, 2021; Energy in Europe, 2022). Because of the integrated nature of the global food system, the war's effects also threaten increases in food prices that will disproportionately affect households, and countries, at the bottom end of the income spectrum (Agricultural commodities: Grainstorm, 2022; UNCTAD, 2022). Even if the Ukrainian war is rapidly ended, the complexity of the supply chains involved means that some of these increases are likely to take years to unwind. In darker scenarios, famine threatens to return to Europe, and expand its reach elsewhere.

Meanwhile, the pandemic has been very good to those near the very top of income and wealth distributions. The *World Inequality Report 2022* observes that: "Between 2021 and 2019, the wealth of the top 0.001% grew by 14%, while average global wealth is estimated to have risen by just 1%. At the top of the top, global billionaire wealth increased by more than 50% between 2019 and 2021" (Chancel et al., 2021, p. 46). Billionaires in the US made especially impressive gains: as of October 2021, their wealth had grown by US\$2.1 trillion during the pandemic as a consequence of rebounding share prices, with some seeing their wealth more than double (Collins, 2021). Almost none of this windfall "trickled down" to workers at firms like Amazon and Wal-Mart, whose owners were among the lucky winners (Kinder & Stateler, 2020). As with other aspects of the pandemic's economic impact, ongoing comparative analyses of the situation in Europe and elsewhere will be valuable. It is fair to say, however, that a further ratcheting up of inequality, as occurred after the financial crisis and driven both by increases in property values and by concentration of share-price wealth among the very richest, is far more likely than any sort of levelling effect.

2.4 Building Back Better? Taxing Issues and the Improbability of Necessary Responses

The World Health Organization's Commission on Social Determinants of Health began its report with an indictment of the "toxic combination of poor social policies and programmes, unfair economic arrangements, and bad politics" (Commission on Social Determinants of Health, 2008, executive summary) that generate unequal exposures, susceptibilities, and vulnerabilities of the sort that were highlighted and magnified by the pandemic. One of the knowledge networks that supported the Commission organized its generic policy recommendations for reducing health inequalities around the three-Rs rubric of "rights, redistribution, and regulation" (Labonté & Schrecker, 2009), borrowed from the work of a now-disbanded Finnish policy research unit (Deacon et al., 2005). Post-pandemic a fourth R must be added—reinvestment—in order at the very least to restore basic capacities for public health threat response that were neglected or abandoned before the pandemic (Garrett, 2019; Sparke & Williams, 2021).[6] Strategic (re-)investment in vastly larger volumes assumes special importance in light of the need to decarbonize economies to address climate change—widely regarded as necessary apart from the pandemic's effects, and a key element of many "build back better" blueprints.

Implementing the four-Rs, perhaps in particular redistribution and reinvestment, would require a direct confrontation with the neoliberal policy playbook succinctly described by innovation scholar Mariana Mazzucato (2022b, p. 11):

> [T]he dominant economic paradigm of the past five decades has justified government "intervention" only in very limited circumstances—to fix market failures while avoiding government failures. Under this framework, goods and services are most efficiently

---

[6] Incredibly, the UK government in April 2022 announced plans to reduce staffing at the Health Security Agency, responsible for pandemic planning and response, by 40% after budget cuts were imposed by the finance ministry (Mason et al., 2022). Disturbing parallels exist between this action and the US Congressional decision described in note 3, above.

produced by private firms operating in a competitive market, and the state should only "intervene" in markets to correct certain identifiable market failures and only in cases where the "intervention" does not cause a government failure.[7]

Mazzucato argues persuasively (Mazzucato, 2022a) that responding to crises like climate change requires a "mission oriented" approach that *shapes* markets rather than merely correcting for market failures (Mazzucato, 2016), with (for example) "the state acting as an investor of first resort (rather than a lender of last resort) and as a funder and regulator with clear direction . . ." As a national-level indication of the requisite scale, a thorough UK National Audit Office (2020) report made clear the "colossal challenge" of achieving "net zero" greenhouse gas emissions by 2050, to which government claims to be committed, citing annual cost estimates equivalent to 1–2% of GDP. Internationally, even shaping the direction of existing expenditures has proved problematic: 91% of the G20 countries' US\$14 trillion stimulus response to the pandemic did not incorporate measures to reduce greenhouse gas emissions, and some countries' plans actually would increase emissions; the European Union's direct commitments, interestingly, were a conspicuous exception (Nahm et al., 2022).

Even before the pandemic the imperative of implementing progressive[8] redistribution in order to reduce health inequalities had been central to many assessments of political plausibility (Mackenbach, 2010; Schrecker, 2017, 2019; Lynch, 2020). It is useful to begin the assessment of post-pandemic prospects with a thoroughly parochial example: the UK government's March 2022 budgetary response to the pressures earlier described. A range of incremental responses included a reduction in the tax on vehicle fuel (fuel duty), after the duty had been frozen for a decade, which had resulted even before the budget in a net reduction in inflation-adjusted terms. (My neighbours with two Range Rovers on their drive were not doubt quite happy.) The effect was the same as if government had committed to writing cheques to motorists, with the size of the cheque directly related to the amount of fuel they used. Non-motorists, of course, received neither cheques nor their equivalent. This is both

---

[7]Mazzucato consistently avoids using the terminology of neoliberalism, although that is clearly what she is talking about; colleagues like Thomas Marois (2021) who likewise write about mechanisms for stimulating innovation do not share that hesitation.

[8]A terminological note: in public finance, the terms "progressive" and "regressive" have a technical, rather than a normative meaning. A progressive tax or tax system is one that is charged at a higher rate or attaches to a larger proportion of a household's resources as one moves up the income or wealth scale. A regressive tax does the reverse. For example, consumption taxes are almost always regressive because lower-income households normally spend a larger proportion of their incomes for immediate needs. An income tax that is charged at an increasing rate on higher incomes is progressive in the absence of deductions available only to the well off, which can be plentiful and vitiate the progressivity of the tax. A progressive expenditure is one the incidence of which is proportionately more generous to households or communities with fewer resources. Although the point is outside the scope of this chapter, for equity purposes it is important to assess the overall progressivity or regressivity of tax and benefit systems combined, which is difficult because of the importance of valuing in-kind services like public education and health care so is seldom done. For a valuable, more detailed discussion, see Byrne (2021), Chap. 6.

regressive and climate-unfriendly. One think tank concluded that the government's suite of tax and benefit policy changes would deliver two-thirds of its benefits to households in the top half of the income distribution; fail to offset high inflation and stagnant or declining real labour incomes; and push 1.3 million people at the bottom of the income scale into "absolute poverty" (Bell et al., 2022).

The UK example is admittedly an extreme one, from a government that was responsible for a decade of austerity and is pathologically committed to the defence of privilege, so limited inferences can be drawn from it. It nevertheless serves as a useful introduction to the domestic politics of public revenues, spending and investment post-pandemic. Implementing the four-Rs, perhaps in particular redistribution and reinvestment, raises inescapable questions of how to finance necessary initiatives as they need to compete with such priorities as the need, demonstrated by the war in Ukraine, for many countries to increase defence spending. In most high-income countries, the pandemic saw an extensively debt-financed end to a decade of austerity that had been economically counterproductive and socially destructive (Krugman, 2015; Horton, 2017). This had the effect of increasing debt-to-GDP ratios, creating constraints on future policy directions. Unless destructive austerity is to be repeated, further worsening inequality—which unfortunately cannot be ruled out, as illustrated by the UK case described earlier—then tax revenues in the post-pandemic world will eventually have to rise, making the issue of what kinds of taxes and who will pay them critical from an equity perspective. The politics of building back better, and equitably, are therefore inseparable from the politics of taxation. The axiom that "tax is not a four-letter word", as the former head of Canada's public service put it following his retirement (Himelfarb & Himelfarb, 2013), should guide serious policy analysis, but is unlikely to do so.

Given the immense increases in wealth and wealth concentration during the pandemic, the issue of wealth taxation in particular merits more attention. It has been argued that the rise in public debt after the financial crisis of 2007–2008 accelerated a shift of power away from citizens and elected governments and towards the investors whose aggregated portfolio preferences constitute the wisdom of "the markets", and whose "confidence" must be maintained whatever the costs in terms of democratic accountabilities (Streeck, 2015, pp. 10–12). With specific reference to post-crisis Europe, the argument further holds that economic and social policy became dominated by the imperatives of a "consolidation state", driven by the need "to make a state attractive for financial investment by making it clear to the financial markets that the state is in a position to service its debt", with austerity as the means to this end and rapid and volatile increases in the cost of borrowing as the price of failure (Streeck, 2015, p. 10). The account is descriptively accurate, and obviously relevant to much higher public debts post-pandemic, but its implication of inevitability must be rejected, as suggested by Piketty's (2014, p. 542) provocative observation that the post-crisis debts of all European countries could have been eliminated by way of a one-time, exceptional tax on private wealth. In a response to the pandemic before the full extent of its effects on wealth concentration became evident, the United Nations Conference on Trade and Development argued that "[in] light of the further increase in inequality resulting from this crisis the case for a wealth tax seems irrefutable" (UNCTAD, 2020, p. x). Indeed, the *Financial Times'* Editorial Board (2020) conceded that wealth taxes would "have to be in the [policy] mix". Yet for the most part, silence on this point has been deafening even in the shrinking number of countries that still have functioning parties on the electoral left. US president Biden's March 2022 legislative proposal to levy a minimum tax on the ultra-rich and to tax unrealized capital gains on financial assets (Kanno-Youngs, 2022) was a striking outlier, although the institutional perversities of the US Senate meant that it stood a minimal chance of success.

It is not difficult to understand the obstacles. Taxing pandemic windfalls even in formal democracies first of all invites conflict with the ultra-rich, whose influence on politics is outsized both within their national boundaries and across them (see e.g., Harrington, 2016; Belton, 2020, Chaps. 14–15; Geoghegan, 2020) and magnified by opportunities for capital flight. Also to be anticipated as a response to potential wealth taxes on pandemic property windfalls is resistance from a much larger stratum of homeowners, including the expanding ranks of owners of multiple properties, who comprise a majority in many jurisdictions and have been newly enriched by the housing price increases described earlier. Depending on where we live they might include many of our academic colleagues. This stratum almost certainly constitutes a decisive political plurality in many countries at the national level, although their numbers and influence might be less significant within sub-national jurisdictions such as major cities with high population densities and tenant populations. Among many hypotheses for future investigation is therefore that if efforts to build back better have any chance of success, their chances are best in jurisdictions with tenant majorities or near-majorities (so less affected by the drive to preserve property wealth) and, in the case of sub-national units, considerable economic and social policy autonomy as well as sufficient territorial scale to discourage the flight of wealth by way of "secession of the successful" (Reich, 1991) to lower-tax neighbouring jurisdictions. The local electoral success of left- and green-leaning mayors in the cities of Montréal (Valérie Plante) and Paris (Anne Hidalgo) may reflect this dynamic, but how many such jurisdictions are there? And do they have access to necessary policy instruments? A further complication is introduced by a deepening schism between the political allegiances of metropolitan and suburban or rural populations that has been observed across Europe (Kenny & Luca, 2021) and elsewhere. The contours of the divide vary among countries and are mediated by political institutions; without engaging in stereotyping, it is important to note that the urban-rural divide can add a further polarizing dimension to the politics of building back better, as demographic and territorial cleavages reinforce one another.

Apart from considerations of socio-economic and health equity, taxation of one sort or another is also central to the future of climate policy: again, tax must not be a four-letter word. Economists are in remarkable agreement that the most effective way of limiting greenhouse gas emissions is to levy a price on carbon emissions sufficient to bring about predictable reductions to whatever level is considered necessary (e.g. High-Level Commission on Carbon Prices, 2017, Chap. 2). As an illustration, and it is only that, International Monetary Fund (IMF) researchers have estimated that a global average carbon price of US$75/ton would be needed by 2030 to achieve the Paris Agreement objective of limiting average global warming to below 2° C, as compared with a recent global average of US$12/ton for the combination of a limited number of explicit carbon prices with existing energy taxes (Black et al., 2021). In other words, the global average price of carbon emissions would have to increase six-fold. A multitude of policy designs to incorporate equity concerns is possible, including not only different carbon prices related to country income level and the nature of fossil fuel use but also alternative internal uses of revenues, such as (for example) direct compensation to low-income households and reinvestment of revenues in decarbonization measures (Parry, 2019; Vogt-Schilb et al., 2019). Indeed for purposes of building back better some such measures would almost certainly be needed (High-Level Commission on Carbon Prices, 2017). From an equity and also a political perspective, important issues arise within national borders about the legitimacy of imposing costs on those least able to afford them; for example, those low-income households whose contribution to global carbon emissions is far less than that of the ultra-rich, in particular (Chancel, 2022). As just one, blindingly obvious illustration: energy-efficient decarbonization of housing, even if owner-occupied, cannot credibly or equitably be financed by the third of the UK population who, according to a major 2011 study at the start of a decade of austerity, were in low-wage or precarious employment with an average of just under £1000 in savings, even before accounting for household debt (Savage et al., 2013). The situation of this stratum is much grimmer now.

Nevertheless, serious discussion of policy choices for equitably distributing the domestic costs of greenhouse gas reduction is not yet occurring in most of the world, raising hard questions about the domestic political viability of carbon pricing (Ball, 2018). The incantation that "[t]he costs of achieving net zero are highly uncertain but the costs of inaction would be far greater" (National Audit Office, 2020, p. 7), however accurate, does not solve problems of equity and feasibility in implementation. Distributions of the costs of action and inaction are very different, with many of the latter manifesting well into the future or outside the borders within which costs are incurred, and (a massive understatement) actors vary widely in the political resources they can deploy to resist or shift the costs. Further exploration would require many additional chapters; as mentioned earlier, more systematic comparative research at the national and sub-national level is needed on the arguments and conjectures raised here. Meanwhile, one must consider the high probability of interacting and increasingly intense crises of inequality (of health outcomes and their economic substrates) and environmental change. In a scene near the end of Ballard's novel, surviving children play with the bones of the less fortunate in the tower block's rooftop sculpture garden . . .

Acknowledgements The editors' comments on an earlier draft of this chapter resulted in substantial improvements. All remaining problems are of my own making.

References

Adkins, L., Cooper, M., & Konings, M. (2021). Class in the 21st century: Asset inflation and the new logic of inequality. *Environment and Planning A: Economy and Space, 53*, 548–572.

Agricultural Commodities: Grainstorm. (2022). March 12. *The Economist*, 65–66.

Alexander, M., Unruh, L., Koval, A., & Belanger, W. (2021). United States response to the COVID-19 pandemic, January-November 2020. *Health Economics, Policy and Law*. https://doi.org/10.1017/S1744133121000116

Arsenault, C., Gage, A., Kim, M. K., Kapoor, N. R., Akweongo, P., Amponsah, F., et al. (2022). COVID-19 and resilience of healthcare systems in ten countries. *Nature Medicine*. https://doi.org/10.1038/s41591-022-01750-1

Baldwin, P. (2021). *Fighting the first wave: Why the Coronavirus was tackled so differently across the globe*. Cambridge University Press.

Ball, J. (2018). Hot air won't Fly: The new climate consensus that carbon pricing isn't cutting it. *Joule, 2*, 2491–2494.

Ballard, J. G. (1975). *High-Rise*. Jonathan Cape.

Bambra, C., Lynch, J., & Smith, K. E. (2021). *The unequal pandemic: Covid-19 and health inequalities*. Policy Press.

Bell, T., Brewer, M., Corlett, A., Hale, S., Handscomb, K., Judge, L., et al. (2022). *Inflation nation: Putting spring statement 2022 in context*. Resolution Foundation. https://www.resolutionfoundation.org/app/uploads/2022/03/Inflation-nation.pdf

Belton, C. (2020). *Putin's people: How the KGB took back Russia and then took on the West*. William Collins.

Bentley, R., Baker, E., & Aitken, Z. (2019). The 'double precarity' of employment insecurity and unaffordable housing and its impact on mental health. *Social Science and Medicine, 225*, 9–16.

Birn, A.-E., Pillay, Y., & Holtz, T. (2017). *Textbook of global health* (4th ed.). Oxford University Press.

Black, S., Parry, I., Roaf, J., & Zhunussova, K. (2021). *Not yet on track to net zero: The urgent need for greater ambition and policy action to achieve Paris temperature goals*, IMF Staff Climate Note 2021/005. International Monetary Fund. https://www.elibrary.imf.org/downloadpdf/journals/066/2021/005/066.2021.issue-005-en.pdf

Blakeley, G. (2021). Financialization, real estate and Covid-19 in the UK. *Community Development Journal, 56*, 79–99.

Bollyky, T. J., Nuzzo, J., Huhn, N., Kiernan, S., & Pond, E. (2022). Global vaccination must be swifter. *Nature, 603*, 788–792.

Brewer, M., & Tasseva, I. (2020). *Did the UK Policy Response to Covid-19 Protect household incomes?* Resolution Foundation and University of Essex. https://doi.org/10.2139/ssrn.3628464

Byrne, D. S. (2021). *Inequality in a context of climate crisis after Covid: A complex realist approach*. Routledge.

Capgemini & Merrill Lynch Wealth Management. (2011). *World wealth report 2011*. Merrill Lynch Global Wealth Management.

Capgemini Research Institute. (2020). *World wealth report 2020*. Capgemini. https://www.capgemini.com/nl-nl/wp-content/uploads/sites/7/2020/07/World-Wealth-Report-WWR-2020.pdf

Chancel, L. (2022). Global carbon inequality, 1990-2019: The impact of wealth concentration on the distribution of world emissions (preprint). *Research Square*. https://www.researchsquare.com/article/rs-1404683/latest.pdf

Chancel, L., Piketty, T., Saez, E., & Zucman, G. (2021). *World inequality report 2022*. World Inequality Lab. https://wir2022.wid.world/www-site/uploads/2021/12/WorldInequalityReport2022_FullReport.pdf

Cheshmehzangi, A. (2022). Vulnerability of the UK's BAME communities during Covid-19: The review of public health and socio-economic inequalities. *Journal of Human Behavior in the Social Environment, 32*, 172–188.

Child Allowance: The Social Experiment. (2022). April 2. *The Economist*, 33–34.

Collins, C. (2021). *Updates: Billionaire wealth, U.S. job losses and pandemic profiteers.* Inequality.org. https://inequality.org/great-divide/updates-billionaire-pandemic/

Comas-Herrera, A., Zalakaín, J., Lemmon, E., Henderson, D., Litwin, C., Hsu, A. T., et al. (2021). *Mortality associated with Covid-19 in care homes: International evidence.* International Long Term Care Policy Network. https://www.longliveheelderly.org/wp-content/uploads/2021/05/LTC_COVID_19_international_report_January-1-February-1-2-1.pdf

Commission on Social Determinants of Health. (2008). *Closing the gap in a generation: Health equity through action on the social determinants of health (final report).* World Health Organization. http://whqlibdoc.who.int/publications/2008/9789241563703_eng.pdf

Covid-19 Excess Mortality Collaborators. (2022). Estimating excess mortality due to the Covid-19 pandemic: A systematic analysis of Covid-19-related mortality, 2020-21. *The Lancet.* https://doi.org/10.1016/S0140-6736(21)02796-3

Deacon, B., Ilva, M., Koivusalo, M., Ollila, E., & Stubbs, P. (2005). *Copenhagen social summit ten years on: The need for effective social policies nationally, regionally and globally.* GASPP Policy Brief No. 6. Globalism and Social Policy Programme, STAKES. https://bib.irb.hr/datoteka/191427.policybrief6.pdf

Diamond, D., & Roubein, R. (2022, April 4). 'Victory for the virus': Senators cut global aid from $10B Covid deal. *Washington Post.*

Dorling, D. (2022). The decimation of the NHS. *The Geographer: Newsletter of the Royal Scottish Geographical Society*, 6–7. https://www.dannydorling.org/?page_id=8808

Energy in Europe: Out of Russia's Shadow. (2022, March 5). *The Economist*, 57–59.

Epstein, G. A. (Ed.). (2005). *Financialization and the world economy.* Edward Elgar.

European Commission. (2019). *The European Green Deal*, COM(2019)640 final. Brussels: European Commission. https://eur-lex.europa.eu/resource.html?uri=cellar:b828d165-1c22-11ea-8c1f-01aa75ed71a1.0002.02/DOC_1&format=PDF

European Commission. (2022). Housing price statistics - house price index. *Eurostat* [On-line]. https://ec.europa.eu/eurostat/statistics-explained/index.php?title=Housing_price_statistics_-_house_price_index

Financial Times Editorial Board. (2020, April 4). Virus lays bare the frailty of the social contract. *Financial Times.*

Flynn, L. B. (2022). The pandemic worsens Europe's housing problems. *Current History, 121*, 83–89.

Freeman, R. B. (2010). It's financialization! *International Labour Review, 149*, 163–183.

Garcia, M. A., Thierry, A. D., & Pendergrast, C. B. (2021). The devastating economic impact of Covid-19 on older black and Latinx adults: Implications for health and well-being. *The Journals of Gerontology: Series B.* https://doi.org/10.1093/geronb/gbab218

Garrett, L. (2019). *The world knows an apocalyptic pandemic is coming.* Foreign Policy.com [On-line]. https://foreignpolicy.com/2019/09/20/the-world-knows-an-apocalyptic-pandemic-is-coming/

Geoghegan, P. (2020). *Democracy for sale: Dark money and dirty politics.* Head of Zeus.

Geronimus, A. T., Hicken, M., Keene, D., & Bound, J. (2006). "Weathering" and age patterns of allostatic load scores among blacks and hites in the United States. *American Journal of Public Health, 96*, 826–833.

Greer, S. L., King, E. J., Massard da Fonseca, E., & Peralta-Santos, A. (Eds.). (2021). *Coronavirus politics: The comparative politics and policy of Covid-19.* University of Michigan Press.

Halimi, S. (2013, May). Tyranny of the one per cent. *Le Monde Diplomatique* (English edition).

Harrington, B. (2016). *Capital without borders: Wealth managers and the one percent.* Harvard University Press.

High-Level Commission on Carbon Prices. (2017). *Report of the high-level commission on carbon prices.* World Bank. https://static1.squarespace.com/static/54ff9c5ce4b0a53decccfb4c/t/59b7f2409f8dce5316811916/1505227332748/CarbonPricing_FullReport.pdf

Himelfarb, A., & Himelfarb, J. (Eds.). (2013). *Tax is not a four letter word: A different take on taxes in Canada*. Wilfrid Laurier University Press.

Horton, R. (2017). Offline: Not one day more. *The Lancet, 390*, 110.

Hughes, R. (2022). *March 2022 Economic and fiscal outlook: Transcript of Presentation*. Office for Budget Responsibility. https://obr.uk/download/economic-and-fiscal-outlook-speaking-notes-march-2022/; https://obr.uk/download/economic-and-fiscal-outlook-presentation-slides-march-2022/

IMF Blog. (2021, October 18). *Housing prices continue to soar in many countries around the world*. IMF Blog [On-line]. https://blogs.imf.org/2021/10/18/housing-prices-continue-to-soar-in-many-countriesaround-the-world/

International Labour Organization. (2012). *Global employment trends 2012: Preventing a deeper jobs crisis*. ILO. https://www.ilo.org/wcmsp5/groups/public/%2D%2D-dgreports/%2D%2D-dcomm/%2D%2D-publ/documents/publication/wcms_171571.pdf

International Labour Organization. (2019). *World employment and social outlook - trends 2019*. ILO. https://www.ilo.org/wcmsp5/groups/public/%2D%2D-dgreports/%2D%2D-dcomm/%2D%2D-publ/documents/publication/wcms_670542.pdf

Jenkins, R. H., Aliabadi, S., Vamos, E. P., Taylor-Robinson, D., Wickham, S., Millett, C., et al. (2021). The relationship between austerity and food insecurity in the UK: A systematic review. *EClinicalMedicine, 33*, 100781.

Kanno-Youngs, Z. (2022, March 27). Tax proposal in budget will target billionaires. *New York Times*, A28.

Kelly, M. P., & Doohan, E. (2012). The social determinants of health. In M. H. Merson, R. E. Black, & A. J. Mills (Eds.), *Global health: Diseases, programs, systems, and policies* (3rd ed., pp. 75–114). Jones & Bartlett Learning.

Kenny, M., & Luca, D. (2021). The urban-rural polarisation of political disenchantment: An investigation of social and political attitudes in 30 European countries. *Cambridge Journal of Regions, Economy and Society, 14*, 565–582.

Kinder, M., & Stateler, L. (2020). *Amazon and Walmart have raked in billions in additional profits during the pandemic, and shared almost none of it with their workers*. Brookings Institution [On-line]. https://www.brookings.edu/blog/the-avenue/2020/12/22/amazon-and-walmart-have-raked-in-billions-in-additional-profits-during-the-pandemic-and-shared-almost-none-of-it-with-their-workers/

Kourti, A., Stavridou, A., Panagouli, E., Psaltopoulou, T., Spiliopoulou, C., Tsolia, M., et al. (2021). Domestic violence during the Covid-19 Pandemic: A systematic review. *Trauma, Violence, & Abuse*. https://doi.org/10.1177/15248380211038690

Krippner, G. R. (2011). *Capitalizing on crisis: The political origins of the rise of finance*. Harvard University Press.

Krugman, P. (2015, April 29). The Austerity Delusion. *Guardian*. http://www.theguardian.com/business/ng-interactive/2015/apr/29/the-austerity-delusion

Labonté, R., & Schrecker, T. (2009). Rights, redistribution, and regulation. In R. Labonté, T. Schrecker, C. Packer, & V. Runnels (Eds.), *Globalization and health: Pathways, evidence and policy* (pp. 317–333). Routledge.

Lynch, J. (2020). *Regimes of inequality: The political economy of health and wealth*. Cambridge University Press.

Mackenbach, J. P. (2010). Has the English strategy to reduce health inequalities failed? *Social Science and Medicine, 71*, 1249–1253.

Marois, T. (2021). *Public banks: Decarbonisation, definancialisation and democratisation*. Cambridge University Press.

Mason, R., Stewart, H., & Campbell, D. (2022, April 26). UK health agency to cut 800 jobs and halt routine Covid testing. *Guardian*. https://www.theguardian.com/society/2022/apr/26/uk-health-agency-to-cut-40-of-jobs-and-suspend-routine-Covid-testing

Mastini, R., Kallis, G., & Hickel, J. (2021). A green new deal without growth? *Ecological Economics, 179*, 106832.

Mazzucato, M. (2016). From market fixing to market-creating: A new framework for innovation policy. *Industry and Innovation, 23*, 140–156.

Mazzucato, M. (2022a). Financing the green new deal. *Nature Sustainability, 5*, 93–94.

Mazzucato, M. (2022b). *Inclusive and sustainable British Columbia: A mission-oriented approach to a renewed economy.* Institute for Innovation and Public Purpose, University College London. https://www.ucl.ac.uk/bartlett/public-purpose/sites/bartlett_public_purpose/files/ucl-iipp-british-columbia-report-2022.pdf

Measuring Poverty: The Hunger Wanes. (2021, June 5). *The Economist.*

Nahm, J. M., Miller, S. M., & Urpelainen, J. (2022). G20's US$14-trillion economic stimulus reneges on emissions pledges. *Nature, 603*, 28–31.

National Audit Office. (2020). *Achieving net zero: Report by the comptroller and auditor general* No. HC1035. NAO. https://www.nao.org.uk/wp-content/uploads/2020/12/Achieving-net-zero.pdf

Nguyen, V.-K. & Kickbusch, I. (2021). *World Health Day 2031: Looking back on the pandemic from the future.* Graduate Institute Geneva. https://www.graduateinstitute.ch/communications/news/world-health-day-2031-looking-back-pandemic-future

OECD (Organisation for Economic Co-operation and Development). (2020a). *Building back better: A sustainable, resilient recovery after Covid-19.* Organisation for Economic Co-operation and Development. https://read.oecd-ilibrary.org/view/?ref=133_133639-s08q2ridhf&title=Building-back-better-_A-sustainable-resilient-recovery-after-Covid-19

OECD (Organisation for Economic Co-operation and Development). (2020b). *Paid sick leave to protect income, health and jobs through the Covid-19 crisis.* OECD. https://read.oecd-ilibrary.org/view/?ref=134_134797-9iq8w1fnju&title=Paid-sick-leave-to-protect-income-health-and-jobs-through-the-COVID-19-crisis

Office for National Statistics. (2021a). *Coronavirus (COVID-19) related deaths by occupation, England and Wales: deaths registered between 9 March and 28 December 2020.* ONS. https://www.ons.gov.uk/peoplepopulationandcommunity/healthandsocialcare/causesofdeath/bulletins/coronavirusCovid19relateddeathsbyoccupationenglandandwales/deathsregisteredbetween9marchand28december2020/pdf

Office for National Statistics. (2021b). *Deaths due to Covid-19 by local area and deprivation.* ONS. https://www.ons.gov.uk/file?uri=%2fpeoplepopulationandcommunity%2fbirthsdeathsandmarriages%2fdeaths%2fdatasets%2fdeathsduetoCovid19bylocalareaanddeprivation%2fapril2021/Covidlocalareadeprivationapril2021.xlsx

Office for National Statistics. (2021c). *EMP17: People in employment on zero hours contracts.* https://www.ons.gov.uk/employmentandlabourmarket/peopleinwork/employmentandemployeetypes/datasets/emp17peopleinemploymentonzerohourscontracts

Office for National Statistics. (2022). *UK House Price Index: December 2021.* ONS. https://www.ons.gov.uk/economy/inflationandpriceindices/bulletins/housepriceindex/december2021

Or, Z., Gandré, C., Durand Zaleski, I., & Steffen, M. (2021). France's response to the Covid-19 pandemic: Between a rock and a hard place. *Health Economics, Policy and Law.* https://doi.org/10.1017/S1744133121000165

Parry, I. (2019, December). Putting a price on pollution. *Finance & Development, 56*, 16–19.

Penne, T., & Goedemé, T. (2021). Can low-income households afford a healthy diet? Insufficient income as a driver of food insecurity in Europe. *Food Policy, 99*, 101978.

Piketty, T. (2014). *Capital in the twenty-first century.* Belknap Press of Harvard University Press.

Piquero, A. R., Jennings, W. G., Jemison, E., Kaukinen, C., & Knaul, F. M. (2021). Evidence from a systematic review and meta-analysis: Domestic violence during the Covid-19 Pandemic. *Journal of Criminal Justice, 74*, 101806.

Pool, U., & Dooris, M. (2021). Prevalence of food security in the UK measured by the Food Insecurity Experience Scale. *Journal of Public Health.* https://doi.org/10.1093/pubmed/fdab120

Prime Cuts. (2019, March 9). *The Economist*, 65–66.

Reich, R. (1991, January 20). Secession of the successful. *New York Times Magazine, 16–17*, 42–45.

Rocha, R., Shingler, B., & Montpetit, J. (2020, June 11). Montreal's poorest and most racially diverse neighbourhoods hit hardest by COVID-19, data analysis shows. *CBC News*. https://www.cbc.ca/news/canada/montreal/race-Covid-19-montreal-data-census-1.5607123

Rolnik, R. (2020). Housing under the empire of finance. In J. Knox-Hayes & D. Wójcik (Eds.), *The routledge handbook of financial geography* (pp. 189–207). Routledge.

Savage, M., Devine, F., Cunningham, N., Taylor, M., Li, Y., Hjellbrekke, J., et al. (2013). A new model of social class? Findings from the BBC's Great British Class Survey Experiment. *Sociology, 47*, 219–250.

Scheidel, W. (2017). *The great leveler: Violence and the history of inequality from the Stone Age to the twenty-first century*. Princeton University Press.

Schrecker, T. (2017). Was Mackenbach right? Towards a practical political science of redistribution and health inequalities. *Health & Place, 46*, 293–299.

Schrecker, T. (2019). The Commission on Social Determinants of Health: Ten years on, a tale of a sinking stone, or of promise yet unrealised? *Critical Public Health, 29*, 610–615.

Schrecker, T. (2021). Neoliberal epidemics: Etiology, a bit of history, and a view from Ground Zero. In J. Gabe, M. Cardano, & A. Genova (Eds.), *Health and illness in the neoliberal era in Europe* (pp. 11–30). Emerald Publishing.

Schrecker, T., & Bambra, C. (2015). *How politics makes us sick: Neoliberal epidemics*. Palgrave Macmillan.

Sparke, M., & Williams, O. D. (2021). Neoliberal disease: Covid-19, co-pathogenesis and global health insecurities. *Environment and Planning A: Economy and Space*. https://doi.org/10.1177/0308518X211048905

Streeck, W. (2015). *The rise of the European Consolidation State*, MPIfG Discussion Paper 15/1. Max Planck Institute for the Study of Societies. http://hdl.handle.net/10419/107091.

Take Your Child to Work (Every) Day. (2021, May 22). The Economist, 54–56.

Tan, R., Harden, J. D., & Brice-Saddler, M. (2022, March 18). The omicron wave's unequal toll. *Washington Post*. https://www.washingtonpost.com/dc-md-va/2022/03/18/dc-Covid-inequality-maryland-virginia/.

The Battle of the Markups. (2022, February 19). *The Economist*.

The Pandemic Is Widening Educational Inequality. (2020, July 27). *The Economist*. https://www.economist.com/graphic-detail/2020/07/27/the-pandemic-is-widening-educational-inequality

The Pandemic's True Death Toll. (2022, March 21; updated daily). *The Economist*. https://www.economist.com/graphic-detail/coronavirus-excess-deaths-estimates

Thelen, K. (2019). The American precariat: U.S. capitalism in comparative perspective. *Perspectives on Politics, 17*, 5–27.

UNCTAD (United Nations Conference on Trade and Development). (2017). *Trade and development report 2017 - Beyond austerity: Towards a global New Deal*. United Nations. http://unctad.org/en/PublicationsLibrary/tdr2017_en.pdf

UNCTAD (United Nations Conference on Trade and Development). (2019). *Trade and development report 2019: Financing a global green new deal*. United Nations. https://unctad.org/en/PublicationsLibrary/tdr2019_en.pdf

UNCTAD (United Nations Conference on Trade and Development). (2020). *Trade and development report 2020: From global pandemic to prosperity for all: Avoiding another lost decade*. United Nations. https://unctad.org/en/PublicationsLibrary/tdr2020_en.pdf

UNCTAD (United Nations Conference on Trade and Development). (2022). The impact on trade and development of the war in Ukraine - *UNCTAD rapid assessment*, UNCTAD/OSG/INF/2022/1. https://unctad.org/system/files/official-document/osginf2022d1_en.pdf

Vampa, D. (2021). Covid-19 and territorial policy dynamics in Western Europe: Comparing France, Spain, Italy, Germany, and the United Kingdom. *Publius*. https://doi.org/10.1093/publius/pjab017

van Loon, J., & Aalbers, M. B. (2017). How real estate became 'just another asset class': The financialization of the investment strategies of Dutch institutional investors. *European Planning Studies, 25*, 221–240.

Vogt-Schilb, A., Walsh, B., Feng, K., Di Capua, L., Liu, Y., Zuluaga, D., et al. (2019). Cash transfers for pro-poor carbon taxes in Latin America and the Caribbean. *Nature Sustainability, 2*, 941–948.

Walker, P. (2022, February 7). Sajid Javid denies row with Treasury behind NHS backlog plan delay. *Guardian*. https://www.theguardian.com/society/2022/feb/07/sajid-javid-denies-row-with-treasury-behind-nhs-backlog-plan-delay

Wallenburg, I., Helderman, J. K., Jeurissen, P., & Bal, R. (2021). Unmasking a health care system: the Dutch policy response to the Covid-19 crisis. *Health Economics, Policy and Law*. https://doi.org/10.1017/S1744133121000128

Wetzstein, S. (2017). The global urban housing affordability crisis. *Urban Studies, 54*, 3159–3177.

What Is Behind Rocketing Natural-Gas Prices? (2021, September 20). *The Economist*. https://www.economist.com/graphic-detail/2021/09/20/what-is-behind-rocketing-natural-gas-prices

Where the Lawns Are Greener. (2022, April 30). *The Economist, 81*.

Ted Schrecker is a Canadian political scientist who relocated to the United Kingdom in 2013 to take up a position as a Professor of Global Health Policy, first at Durham University and (since 2017) at Newcastle University. He is Emeritus Professor as of October 2022. His research interests focus on the political economy of health inequalities, on multiple scales, as they are affected by neoliberal globalization, and on the politics of the evidence–policy interface. His work has been published in journals such as *Critical Public Health, Global Public Health, Globalization and Health, Health & Place, Health Policy & Planning, Medicine Anthropology Theory, Review of International Political Economy, Social Science and Medicine*, and *Sociology Compass*. From 2005 to 2008, he coordinated the knowledge network on globalization that supported the work of the WHO Commission on Social Determinants of Health, and from 2014–2019, he was co-editor of the *Journal of Public Health*.

Chapter 3
The Economic Repercussions of Covid-19 and Well-Being in Georgia

Kakhaber-George Lazarashvili, David Sikharulidze, Tamta Lekishvili, and Vasil Kikutadze

Abstract In this chapter, the impact of the Covid-19 pandemic on certain sectors of the Georgian economy, which in turn has affected unemployment and well-being, will be studied. On the one hand, the paper will investigate the effects of decisions and policies implemented during the pandemic by the Georgian government. By analysing the policy documents, assessments, and statements of officials from the Georgian government, the effectiveness of those decisions in terms of inequalities and thus well-being will be assessed. On the other hand, a relationship between the Covid-19 pandemic and the unemployment rate during 2020 and 2021 in the Caucasus (Georgia, Azerbaijan, and Armenia) countries is empirically examined. Variables such as Covid-19 cases, lockdown, and income support are considered. For the purpose of inference, the paper employs a linear regression model. Findings show that the impact of Covid-19 cases on the unemployment rate is positive, although not statistically significant, lockdown has a positive impact on unemployment growth (increased unemployment rate) and this variable is statistically significant, and government support has a negative impact on unemployment growth.

3.1 Introduction

On 31 December 2019, a novel coronavirus was detected in the city of Wuhan, Hubei Province, which was reported to the World Health Organization (WHO) China Office (WHO, 2020). The virus quickly became a major global health crisis (Li et al., 2020). On January 30, 2020, the WHO declared a new virus a public health emergency (Zhang & Shaw, 2020). The International Committee on Taxonomy of Viruses (ICTV) described the new virus on February 11, 2020 as, a serious acute coronavirus syndrome (SARS-CoV-2), now referred to as "Covid-19" by the WHO

K.-G. Lazarashvili (✉) · D. Sikharulidze · T. Lekishvili · V. Kikutadze
East European University (EEU), Tbilisi, Georgia
e-mail: k.lazarashvili@eeu.edu.ge; d.sikharulidze@eeu.edu.ge; t.lekishvili@eeu.edu.ge;
v.kikutadze@eeu.edu.ge

© The Author(s), under exclusive license to Springer Nature Switzerland AG 2022   41
L. Dalingwater et al. (eds.), *The Unequal Costs of Covid-19 on Well-being in Europe*,
Human Well-Being Research and Policy Making,
https://doi.org/10.1007/978-3-031-14425-7_3

(Sharma et al., 2020). The World Health Organization declared the coronavirus disease a global pandemic on March 11, 2020 (Li et al., 2020).

After the first case of Covid-19 was detected in Georgia in February 2020, from March 21st to the end of May, a state of emergency was declared throughout the country, economic restrictions were imposed, and a number of economic activities were restricted, and borders were closed. The global pandemic has led to a significant decline in revenues from export and international travel, remittances and inflows of foreign direct investment.

Risks from the global macro-financial environment, such as declining global demand, rising risks in developing countries, travel uncertainty and remittances, will negatively affect Georgia's balance of payments inflows and economic growth in the near future.

The spread of the virus has hampered the continuation of the trends observed in the previous years in various directions of the country's economy. In particular, in 2019, economic growth was recorded at 5.1%. Revenue generated from tourism in the country's economy amounted to $ 3.3 billion (18.4% of GDP), revenue from exports of goods: $ 3.8 billion (21.2% of GDP), while net remittances:$1.5 billion (8.4% of GDP). As a result, the country's current account deficit was 5.1% of GDP. Despite these positive economic indicators, the shock of the coronavirus pandemic significantly worsened Georgia's economic growth prospects for 2020 (National Statistics Office of Georgia, 2022).

Risks caused by the pandemic in the international macro-financial environment will be transmitted to Georgia's financial stability through several key channels. Restrictions imposed to prevent the rapid spread of the Covid-19 virus have negatively affected the inflow of international financial flows. In particular, the restriction of international air traffic in the first two quarters of 2020 significantly reduced the number of international visitors and revenues from international travel.

At the same time, economic hardships in trading partner countries have reduced remittances and exports of goods and services. Also, as a result of the increase in risk premiums in countries with growing economies, financial conditions have tightened, which, despite the decline in global interest rates, has led to an increase in foreign currency loans on the supply side. All this was reflected in a significant decrease in financial inflows, which in turn led to the devaluation of the local currency and increased exchange rate fluctuations.

The rest of the paper is organized as follows: In part 2, we review the relevant literature on this topic; part 3 describes the data used and the estimation method, part 4 focuses on the stylized facts about the labour market in Georgia during pandemic and elaborates results; part 5 relates the conclusions of this research.

3.2 Literature Review

The economic crisis can be defined as a phase of the reproduction cycle during which the economy faces difficulties for a long time. Macroeconomic indicators are falling sharply, manifested by declining production and demand, disruption of existing industrial relations, rising unemployment and bankruptcy of businesses, which automatically leads to an increase in poverty and a decline in the living standards of the population.

The negative impact of events such as pandemics, epidemics, and natural disasters on macroeconomic variables is not a new phenomenon. Numerous studies in this area have been conducted, for example, by Fasanya et al. (2020), McKibbin & Fernando (2021). These studies reveal that the effects of the pandemic extend to various sectors such as travel, tourism, and supply chain management. It also causes stock market volatility and oil price fluctuations (Fairlie, 2020).

As a result of the pandemic, the international movement of goods (export–import) has suffered significant delays. Economic activity has declined around the world due to declining travel (Ji, 2020; Vanov, 2020). Panic among consumers and firms has significantly damaged established patterns of consumption of goods and services and created certain anomalies in commodity markets (Baker et al., 2020). Covid-19 has posed significant challenges to the world economy due to the accelerating spread of the virus and has affected almost all sectors of the economy (Demertzis et al., 2020).

The damage caused by the Covid-19 pandemic crisis to the country's economy and human well-being is irreversible and growing. Measures were taken to prevent the spread of the pandemic and to save human lives, in particular: the closure of international and national borders, the declaration of a state of emergency, and the restriction of economic activities due to the virus have dealt a significant blow to the economies of the world (Haryanto, 2020; Kartseva & Kuznetsova, 2020) including Georgia (Ordinance of the Government of Georgia, 2020). The vulnerable groups especially affected are in the tourism sector, such as tour operators, hotels, restaurants, transport, or tour companies, which depend on foreign visitors and create a expanding and inclusive economy. The pandemic also caused significant damage to the retail, transport, construction, manufacturing, real estate, leisure, and entertainment sectors. This situation has had a direct impact on the labour market and labour relations. In particular, the management of the firm was forced to pay salaries to employees with delays and violations of labour rights such as: dismissal without notice; refusal to provide employees with salaries and compensation provided by law at the time of dismissal; refusal to pay compensation during periods of temporary incapacity for work, including quarantine or self-isolation; refusal to provide employees with salaries and compensation provided by law at the time of dismissal (Chanturidze & Surmava, 2021).

Su et al. (2021) found a strong positive significant correlation between Covid-19 cases and unemployment during the pandemic in some European countries. Although the pandemic had a negative impact on the country's economy, the same cannot be said of lockdowns (Correia et al., 2020). Lockdown may have indirect economic benefits from imposing restrictions on coordinated pandemic management and it can prevent a worse economic downturn. This view is shared by various scholars. In particular, restrictions imposed by governments in 2020 reduced disease transmission without further significant economic delays (Andersen et al., 2020; Lin & Meissner, 2020). Francisco Lhano and Hugo Fonseca note in their paper that lockdown does not have a statistically significant effect on changes in the unemployment rate. In particular, the number of days in lockdown did not affect the labour market, as its characteristics were more important than the length of the economic activities' closure (Lhano & Fonseca, 2021).

In addition, the sectors of the country's economy were asymmetrically affected during the pandemic period and the unemployment rate also varies between these sectors. Lockdown has had a different impact on people depending on the field of work. Whereas some work areas allowed people to work remotely thus reducing the negative effects of the pandemic. The negative effects of the pandemic could be reduced for people working in some areas such as education, communication, health care equipment and supplies, life science tools and services, pharmaceuticals, etc.

Regarding social problems, the findings showed that the higher the level of education, the greater the chance of getting a job and maintaining employee status in a labour market crisis. That is to say, better-educated people tend to have lower unemployment because, on a regular basis, the unemployment rate decreases with increasing qualification levels (Bowles & Gintis, 2001), while the least skilled workers are most vulnerable to unemployment during the economic downturn (Gangl, 2001).

According to the International Labor Organization (ILO), in the second quarter of 2020, compared to the fourth quarter of 2019, total reduced working hours amounted to about 400 million lost jobs, which is much more than the 155 million lost jobs in the first quarter. The effects of the pandemic, and subsequent restrictions on women employed in the informal sector, were particularly and disproportionately severe. According to the International Labor Organization, globally 42% of informally employed women work in sectors severely affected by the pandemic.

The Covid-19 crisis has had an unequal impact on employment prospects and incomes across different groups of employees. Young workers, workers with low levels of education, on low-paying jobs and fixed-term contracts have been more likely to experience job or income loss after the onset of a crisis (Adams-Prassl et al., 2020; Elliot & Stephen, 2018).

3.3   Research Methodology

A framework of analysis to determine the effects of the Covid-19 pandemic on the unemployment rate between 2020 and 2021 in Caucasus (Georgia, Azerbaijan, and Armenia) countries was used. Specified model for Covid-19 pandemic impact and the expected signs of the coefficients of regressors are as follows (Elliott et al., 1996):

Table 3.1 Variables of the equation

Variable	Description	Source
UnempRate	**Unemployment rate, percent in Country.**	International Labour Organization
CaseCOVID	Quarterly new confirmed Covid-19 cases	Our world in data
Lockdown	The stringency index—The nine metrics used to calculate the Stringency Index are: school closures; workplace closures; cancellation of public events; restrictions on public gatherings; closures of public transport; stay-at-home requirements; public information campaigns; restrictions on internal movements; and international travel controls. The index on any given day is calculated as the mean score of the nine metrics, each taking a value between 0 and 100. A higher score indicates a stricter response (i.e. 100 = strictest response).	Our world in data
Income support	Income support during the Covid-19 pandemic (income support captures if the government covered the salaries or provided direct cash payments, universal basic income, or similar, of people who lost their jobs or were unable to work).	Our world in data

$$\text{Unemrate} = \beta_0 + \beta_1 \text{CaseCOVID}_t + \varepsilon_t$$

$$\text{Unemrate} = \beta_0 + \beta_1 \text{Lockdown}_t + \varepsilon_t$$

Additionally, both Covid-19 related variables are regressed in the same baseline model, to which variables will be thereafter added:

$$\text{Unemrate} = \beta_0 + \beta_1 \text{CaseCOVID}_t + \beta_2 \text{Lockdown}_t + \beta_3 \text{Incomesupport}_t + \varepsilon_t$$

$\beta_0, \beta_1, \beta_2 = $ *parameters to be estimated,*
$t = 1, \ldots, T = $ *the period of time, quarterly,*
$\varepsilon_t = $ white noise error term.
The variables appearing in the equations are defined as follows (Table 3.1):

3.4   Research Findings

Like other countries in the world, Georgia has also experienced an economic recession caused by the Covid-19 pandemic. The economic effects of the pandemic were caused by the ongoing processes in the world economy, in particular, the reduction of international capital movements, reduced international travel, delayed international movement of goods, reduced remittances, and the decision of the government to declare the lockdown. The Georgian government made a decision on lockdown in the spring and fall of 2020. These developments were reflected in the country's macroeconomic indicators, including the unemployment rate. Thus, this section presents the impact of the pandemic, namely, on the one hand, the impact of ongoing processes in the world economy on the Georgian economy, and on the other hand, the impact of government decisions made during the pandemic on the unemployment rate.

First, we start with macroeconomic analysis. In the second quarter of 2020, GDP decreased by 12.3%, compared to the same period last year, while in the third quarter it decreased even more and amounted to −5.6%. This was due to the fact that the second quarter of 2020 was the lockdown period, as a result of which the decline mostly affected areas such as: administrative and support service activities (−54.7%); Accommodation and food delivery activities (−40%); Professional, scientific, and technical activities (−28.8%); Construction (−24.5%); Art, entertainment, and leisure (−24.1%); Transport and warehousing (−22.6%); Financial and insurance activities (−15.5%); Repair of automobiles and motorcycles (−13.2%), Manufacturing (−12.1%) (Table 3.2).

Growth was observed in the following sectors: health and social services (14.3%), education (11.7%), agriculture, forestry, and fisheries (4.7%), and mining (6.4%).

In the third quarter of 2020, the structure of the economic downturn has partially changed—a small increase in construction was observed (2%); The largest declines were in accommodation and catering activities—same as tourism (−53.1%); Transport and warehousing (−25%), arts, entertainment, and leisure (−32.4%)—the last two areas are related to tourism.

In the fourth quarter of 2020, real GDP fell by 6.8% compared to the same period last year. This decline was due to the decline in economic activity, both within the country and due to the spread of the Covid-19 pandemic in the region. In 2020, real GDP growth was set at −6.2%. The negative effects of the Covid-19 pandemic began in the first quarter of 2020. The number of visits from abroad began to decline in February, and in March, due to the declaration of state of emergency and the closure of borders, revenues from tourism were almost zero.

Consequently, the output of the tourism industry, which is related to other sectors, and has been a large (10–12%) part of the economy in recent years, significantly decreased in 2020. Over the years, the share of tourism in the Georgian economy has grown at a high rate, which has made the economy significantly dependent on this sector. The tourism sector has been hit hard by the pandemic and has shrunk by almost 100%. In 2020, in real terms, there was a significant decline in the sectors of accommodation and food supply (−37.9% ann.), transport and warehousing (−22.3% ann.), trade (−5.6% ann.), construction (4.7% ann.) in the arts, entertainment, and leisure (−18.9% ann.) sectors. The crisis has had little impact on the industrial and agricultural sectors. Real growth was observed in agriculture (+3.6% ann.), health and social services (+7.9% ann.), and education (+3.1% ann.). 2021 also started with a negative economic growth rate due to foreign travel and social distancing measures within the country (National Statistics Office of Georgia).

During 2020, the dynamics of the inflation rate was under significant pressure from both supply and demand. Restrictions due to the spread of the Covid-19 virus complicated and slowed down production, which led to increased costs, which in

Table 3.2 Real gross domestic product growth rates

Economic activities	I 19	II 19	III 19	IV 19	2019	I 20	II 20	III 20	IV 20	2020	I 21*	II 21*	III 21*	IV 21*	2021*
Agriculture, forestry, and fishing	96.2	103.7	104.1	96.5	100.7	102.7	117.7	102.1	107.5	108.1	100.2	96.6	97.1	101.9	98.6
Mining and quarrying	106.6	106.0	103.2	117.3	108.2	113.2	117.7	114.4	105.8	112.4	148.3	115.9	102.2	101.6	113.5
Manufacturing	98.0	95.6	102.8	107.4	101.3	110.1	89.3	92.6	85.1	92.9	97.0	136.2	107.3	100.2	109.0
Electricity, gas, steam and air conditioning supply	104.1	114.5	100.1	102.3	105.3	93.6	97.9	91.1	96.8	94.8	90.6	116.1	178.8	156.5	133.5
Water supply; sewerage, waste management and remediation activities	107.7	123.5	126.4	128.1	121.5	89.0	72.1	73.9	76.6	77.5	124.3	143.4	135.1	154.5	138.9
Construction	91.5	95.1	106.9	105.0	100.7	117.6	66.0	93.0	97.3	92.0	77.9	117.2	70.3	66.6	78.2
Wholesale and retail trade; repair of motor vehicles and motorcycles	104.5	105.5	109.8	112.2	108.3	102.4	78.8	101.9	97.8	95.3	106.2	158.9	112.3	111.2	119.9
Transportation and storage	110.3	110.2	103.7	110.0	108.4	100.0	70.8	70.2	72.1	77.0	94.1	145.5	129.0	140.6	127.6
Accommodation and food service activities	119.3	116.6	117.8	120.5	118.5	98.3	43.1	47.4	43.7	55.1	49.9	199.4	149.8	172.8	129.8
Information and communication	119.1	120.3	123.8	122.0	121.4	107.7	88.0	105.7	108.3	102.6	118.1	151.0	118.4	114.4	123.9
Financial and insurance activities	102.1	93.4	92.5	84.1	92.5	93.2	86.8	97.3	113.1	97.7	123.8	145.0	120.3	110.1	123.5
Real estate activities	106.6	105.4	101.9	102.8	104.1	103.2	95.7	99.5	100.6	99.7	95.9	119.7	106.6	115.0	109.2
Professional, scientific, and technical activities	115.3	112.2	107.3	96.8	107.1	88.0	78.3	91.6	86.9	86.2	99.9	124.8	109.4	106.3	109.8
Administrative and support service activities	123.8	115.3	106.5	108.5	112.5	87.0	44.7	44.5	50.9	54.8	63.7	107.4	140.8	127.9	105.6

(continued)

Table 3.2 (continued)

Economic activities	I 19	II 19	III 19	IV 19	2019	I 20	II 20	III 20	IV 20	2020	I 21*	II 21*	III 21*	IV 21*	2021*
Public administration and defence; compulsory social security	101.1	99.4	98.2	95.5	98.4	105.9	100.3	104.8	98.8	102.3	101.6	100.4	96.1	98.5	99.1
Education	112.9	103.4	100.2	103.7	104.9	112.5	116.0	105.2	100.9	108.6	95.1	98.8	92.2	104.4	97.7
Human health and social work activities	105.1	106.3	100.8	115.3	106.8	105.2	103.8	101.5	100.9	102.8	112.2	143.7	123.8	134.4	128.7
Arts, entertainment, and recreation	109.9	122.4	131.5	123.9	122.1	119.0	56.4	78.3	78.1	81.6	75.9	281.0	148.1	131.0	143.1
Other service activities	83.5	88.6	91.0	87.8	87.7	101.7	74.3	79.6	79.4	83.4	60.3	129.6	127.3	129.4	110.3
Activities of households as employers; undifferentiated goods and servicies produc-ing activities of household for own use	154.7	134.5	95.4	86.1	118.1	100.2	95.8	128.9	174.0	119.3	89.0	99.3	70.7	63.9	79.9
(=) GDP at basic prices	104.7	104.5	105.4	105.7	105.1	104.0	86.4	92.3	92.7	93.4	97.1	131.5	109.1	109.4	111.5
(+) Taxes on products	109.1	107.1	105.0	97.9	104.2	97.3	80.7	99.3	92.8	92.5	87.4	108.1	108.4	104.3	102.6
(−) Subsidies on products	102.2	109.4	107.6	103.1	105.8	100.3	108.0	107.7	104.5	105.5	101.0	105.0	100.9	97.3	101.3
(=) GDP at market prices	105.2	104.8	105.4	104.6	105.0	103.3	85.5	93.2	92.6	93.2	95.9	128.9	109.1	108.8	110.4

Source: National Statistics Office, Georgia

Table 3.3 Working hours lost due to the Covid-19 crisis—ILO modelled estimates (%)—Annually

Year	Georgia	Azerbaijan	Armenia
2020	13.5	12	14.9
2021	2.5	4.6	3.5
2022	−0.4	1.2	0.9

Source: ILOSTAT explorer

turn affected the price of the final product. In addition, the depreciation of the existing local currency, the Georgian Lari (GEL) increased the costs of firms that have loans in foreign currency, which, together with imported inflation, leads to higher inflation. As a result of increased production costs and the depreciation of the GEL exchange rate under the pandemic, annual inflation in the second quarter of 2021 was 8.3% (National Statistics Office of Georgia).

Falling production and rising prices have affected the functioning of the labour market. Job losses and reduced working hours as cost-cutting measures were observed in almost all industries, which affected unemployment levels in 2020 and 2021 (Table 3.3).

The unemployment rate in 2020 was 18.5%, which is 0.9% higher than in 2019. The employment rate also fell by 1.5% to 41.1%. 31.9% of the employed are self-employed, while 68.1% wee the employed workforce, whose activity rate was also reduced by 1.3% to 50.5%. Unemployment rate counted 20.4% in the fourth quarter of 2020, 3.5% more than in the previous quarter. In particular, unemployment was 22.2% in urban areas (+5.6% ann.) and 17.7% in rural areas (+1% ann.). The highest unemployment rates were in the 15–24 and 25–34 age groups. In the fourth quarter of 2020, the economically active population accounted for 50% of the working-age population (15 years and older). In the fourth quarter of 2020, the unemployment rate for women was 17.8%, while for men, it was 22.4%.

The level of employment in the fourth quarter of 2020 decreased by 2.3% compared to the corresponding period of 2019. As a result, productivity (ratio of real output to the number of employees) decreased by 0.7% annually. At the same time, the average nominal wage of employees decreased by 0.4%, amounting to 1314 GEL (approximately $450) as of the fourth quarter of 2020 (National Statistics Office of Georgia).

Women in Georgia have a 36.2% lower salary than men. By 2020, 42,000 had lost their jobs. It is noteworthy that most of the unemployed were women. Out of 54,000 reduced jobs, 42,000 (77.7%) came from jobs that employed women (National Statistics Office of Georgia) (Table 3.4).

Although the number of employed women decreased by 42,000, according to National Statistics Office Georgia (Geostat) the number of unemployed women did not increase and on the contrary, decreased by even 6100 while unemployment among men increased by 11,100. This indicates that women, despite losing their jobs, were no longer looking for a new job. Their already low level of economic activity decreased from 43.1% to 40.4%. One of the reasons for the decline in the level of economic activity of women was the increased volume of domestic affairs, especially in childcare activities, as educational institutions went online and

K.-G. Lazarashvili et al.

Table 3.4 Labour force indicators by sex

Man	3Q_2019	4Q_2019	1Q_2020	2Q_2020	3Q_2020	4Q_2020	1Q_2021	2Q_2021	3Q_2021	4Q_2021
Labour force	879.9	861.6	875.4	859.6	877.4	871.7	834.9	900.5	910.4	878.9
Employed	726.2	709.7	693.2	698.1	711.8	676.8	633.7	680.1	712.4	697.7
Hired	465.3	448.3	441.5	430.5	436.4	408.2	388.9	417.0	440.0	413.0
Self-employed	260.6	260.9	251.0	267.1	274.7	267.9	243.5	262.1	271.6	284.3
Not-identified worker	0.3	0.4	0.7	0.5	0.7	0.7	1.2	1.0	0.7	0.4
Unemployed	153.7	151.9	182.2	161.5	165.6	194.9	201.2	220.4	198.0	181.2
Population outside the labour force	545.1	562.8	529.4	532.3	539.1	533.4	556.5	512.6	496.0	513.9
Unemployment rate, percentage	17.5	17.6	20.8	18.8	18.9	22.4	24.1	24.5	21.7	20.6
Labour force participation rate, percentage	61.7	60.5	62.3	61.8	61.9	62.0	60.0	63.7	64.7	63.1
Employment rate, percentage	51.0	49.8	49.3	50.2	50.2	48.2	45.5	48.1	50.7	50.1

Source: National Statistics Office of Georgia

kindergartens were closed. Women were forced to stay at home and engage in household activities.

It can be said that the sectors where women are usually employed have suffered the most as a result of the crisis. Examples are the service sector—hotels, restaurants, and trade sector. Women employed in households—housekeepers, nannies, caregivers, cooks, etc.—also remained unemployed.

The crisis has once again exposed a gender inequality in the labour market. The problem, which was already acute, was exacerbated by more women leaving the workforce and moving into family affairs. It is important for the state to pay more attention to the issue of gender equality, thus reducing the vulnerability of women in the labour market. Steps to reduce gender inequality could include: reasonable pay for maternity leave, guarantees of family and job balancing, investments in care economics, and full pay for maternity leave (Table 3.5).By 2020, construction (16,200) was the sector where the highest number of jobs were lost, followed by the provision of accommodation (12,800) and education (7500). If we evaluate this indicator as a percentage, the biggest loss of 26.3% is observed in the provision of accommodation and catering activities, which is explained by the minimization of tourist flows and restrictions related to the restaurant business. A 16.3% decrease in the workforce was recorded in real estate activities, while the number of employees in the construction sector decreased by 16% (National Statistics Office of Georgia) (Table 3.6).

One of the categories affected by this crisis is the self-employed and the informally employed, which are mainly related to micro and small businesses in Georgia, and, namely, family businesses. As a result of market research (Leka, 2020), family business owners regularly receive money from their business, almost every week. This means that the daily expenses of the family are provided by the income received from the turnover of the business. As a result, during this pandemic, the closure of activities or part-time work, in conditions of tight demand, is reflected in the income of living expenses of these families, which has the effect of reducing their quality of life.

According to Geostat, the informally employed accounts for 34.7% of the total employment, which is a particularly high rate, while the share of the self-employed, according to the new methodology used by Geostat, is 30.7% of the employed. Informal employees are most often found in the following areas: construction; trade, repair of automobiles and household goods; transport; education; providing personal services, employment in family farms, etc.

The crisis has clearly revealed the problems that informal employees face or may encounter. The state compensation that the self-employed received was one-off unlike the hired workers for whom the compensation was issued for 6 months. In total, the compensation of hired workers was 4 times higher than the compensation of the self-employed.

Informally employed people do not meet minimum labour standards, do not enjoy the rights set out in labour law, and do not have social security guarantees.

Most of the self-employed who lost their income were likely to be employed in the non-agricultural sector. A total of 250,000 self-employed people were registered

Table 3.5 Labour force indicators by sex

Woman	3Q_2019	4Q_2019	1Q_2020	2Q_2020	3Q_2020	4Q_2020	1Q_2021	2Q_2021	3Q_2021	4Q_2021
Labour force	696.3	670.2	669.8	655.4	651.5	634.0	612.4	658.6	681.6	657.2
Employed	585.1	567.3	569.5	539.5	557.3	521.1	496.1	534.4	568.8	546.5
Hired	438.9	431.3	449.6	409.1	408.9	396.9	393.9	414.7	421.8	428.1
Self-employed	146.2	135.9	119.8	130.5	148.4	124.0	102.2	119.7	146.9	118.1
Not-identified worker	0.0	0.0	0.0	0.0	0.0	0.2	0.0	0.0	0.0	0.2
Unemployed	111.2	103.0	100.3	115.9	94.1	112.9	116.3	124.2	112.8	110.7
Population outside the labour force	922.8	937.2	938.4	965.7	968.8	972.2	991.1	960.3	925.0	951.2
Unemployment rate, percentage	16.0	15.4	15.0	17.7	14.5	17.8	19.0	18.9	16.6	16.8
Labour force participation rate, percentage	43.0	41.7	41.6	40.4	40.2	39.5	38.2	40.7	42.4	40.9
Employment rate, percentage	36.1	35.3	35.4	33.3	34.4	32.4	30.9	33.0	35.4	34.0

Source: National Statistics Office of Georgia

Table 3.6 Distribution of employed persons by economic activity

	2018	2018	2019	2019	2020	2020
Total	1296.2	0.7	1295.9	−0.03	1241.8	−4.17
Agriculture, forestry, and fishing	253.9	−12.3	247.4	−2.53	246.3	−0.47
Industry	153.9	0.0	147.0	−4.45	141.3	−3.92
Construction	98.8	17.3	101.4	2.67	85.2	−15.97
Wholesale and retail trade; repair of motor vehicles and motorcycles	185.0	5.9	195.9	5.86	188.0	−4.01
Transportation and storage	78.2	11.5	82.0	4.87	79.1	−3.49
Accommodation and food service activities	44.3	16.9	48.8	10.14	36.0	−26.26
Information and communication	20.9	−3.9	19.0	−8.81	19.7	3.63
Financial and insurance activities	33.7	7.9	30.7	−8.89	29.9	−2.74
Real estate activities	4.4	43.8	3.9	−11.90	3.2	−16.29
Professional, scientific, and technical activities	21.2	−3.6	19.0	−10.51	19.2	0.90
Administrative and support service activities	21.3	15.2	22.4	4.92	19.6	−12.58
Public administration and defence; compulsory social security	91.3	1.7	93.2	1.97	94.5	1.43
Education	155.1	−2.6	153.4	−1.10	145.8	−4.92
Human health and social work activities	65.3	−4.0	60.2	−7.77	62.0	2.88
Arts, entertainment, and recreation	28.4	5.8	29.9	5.19	30.0	0.43
Other service activities	20.0	−4.9	22.0	10.05	25.0	13.48
Activities of households as employers; Undifferentiated goods and services-producing activities of households for own use	19.4	34.2	17.9	−7.73	15.0	−15.95

Source: National Statistics Office of Georgia

to receive state compensation. Up to 100,000 of them received compensation fairly quickly (May–June), indicating that these individuals were registered with the Revenue Service. The applications of the remaining 150,000 citizens were considered individually (National Statistics Office of Georgia).

3.5 Analysis of the Impact on Labour Market Slack

Unemployment rates were estimated on a quarterly basis in 2020 and 2021. Carried out when analysing the number of people infected with the virus begins, as well as in the days when people were forced to stay home because of lockdown orders.

Unemployment rates were estimated in 2019 and 2020 on a quarterly basis. When the virus started to spread, a quarantine was declared and people were forced to stay at home.

Table 3.7 shows the impact of the pandemic on employment, in particular the unemployment rate. According to the first model, the impact of Covid-19 cases on the unemployment rate is positive, although not statistically significant. In addition, the constant is significant at a 1% level, suggesting that unemployment increased on average 8.1% in the absence of people reported with the virus, ceteris paribus. According to the second model, the lockdown had a positive effect on the growth of unemployment and this variable is statistically significant. According to the third model, government support had a negative impact on the growth of unemployment, which means that the measures taken by the government during the pandemic to some extent limited the growth of unemployment. However, this variable is not statistically significant.

3.6   Conclusion

After the first case of Covid-19 was detected in Georgia in February 2020, the spread of the virus became irreversible. The pandemic has hampered the continuation of the positive trends observed in the previous years in various areas of the country's economy. In 2020, the unemployment rate in the country reached "a historical maximum" of 18.5%, thus reducing the country's GDP by 6.8%, while the average nominal wage of the employed population was only 1314 GEL ($445). The decline in incomes was particularly severe on low-income families, so their socio-economic situation has worsened and they have become even poorer than they were before the pandemic. Naturally, this situation has reduced the welfare of the country's population and significantly affected the country's tourism, trade, transport, construction, industry, leisure, and entertainment industries and the people employed in them. Companies have massively laid off employees so that most of them have not even received the compensation provided by the country's legislation. Particularly in a difficult situation were the self-employed persons, in which case the compensation paid to them by the state was 4 times less than the compensation paid to the hired persons. Based on a regression analysis conducted in the study, it was found that the impact of Covid-19 cases on the unemployment rate is positive, although not statistically significant, Lockdown has a positive impact on unemployment growth (increased unemployment rate) and this variable is statistically significant, and government support has a negative impact on unemployment growth. The crisis has once again exposed a gender inequality in the labour market. The problem, which was already acute, was exacerbated by more women leaving the workforce and moving into family affairs. Measures taken by the government have to some extent limited the process of increasing unemployment and reducing the welfare of the population.

Table 3.7 Variation of the unemployment rate regressed on the Covid-19 variables

	I		II		III		IV	
	OLS	GLS	OLS	GLS	OLS	GLS	OLS	GLS
Cases Covid	1.28E-08 (9.33E-09)	5.14E-09 (7.05E-09)					1.27E-08 (9.35E-09)	5.36E-09 (5.65E-09)
Lockdown			0.044967 (0.031219)	0.040147*** (0.013058)			0.053725 (0.035193)	0.046919*** (0.01389)
Income supports					−0.010754 (0.712697)	−0.264917 (0.259082)	−0.515723 (0.782210)	−0.308862 (0.250347)
C	7.802670 (2.703583)	8.108109*** (0.292082)	5.848136*** (2.916497)	6.146304*** (0.715136)	8.217029*** (2.724897)	0.722639*** (0.689620)	5.414120*** (4.427288)	5.862401*** (0.741074)
Observations	48	48	48	48	48	48	48	48
R-squared	0.040139	0.711440	0.043839	0.717920	0.000005	0.722639	0.092967	0.736506
Adjusted R-squared	0.019273	0.677088	0.023053	0.684339	−0.021734	0.689620	0.031124	0.690394

Notes: $*p < 0.1$; $**p < 0.05$; $***p < 0.01$

References

Adams-Prassl, A., Boneva, T., Golin, M., & Rauh, C. (2020, April 08). *The large and unequal impact of COVID-19*. Retrieved from VOXEU CEPR: https://voxeu.org/article/large-and-unequal-impact-covid-19-workers

Andersen, A. L., Hansen, E. T., Johannesen, N., & Sheridan , A. (2020). *Pandemic, shutdown and consumer spending: Lessons from scandinavian policy responses to covid-19*. Cornell University. https://arxiv.org/pdf/2005.04630.pdf

Baker, S. R., Bloom, N., Davis, S. J., Kost, K., Sammon, M., & Viratyosin, T. (2020). The unprecedented stock market reaction to Covid-19. *The Review of Asset Pricing Studies* (pp. 742–758). https://academic.oup.com/raps/article/10/4/742/5873533

Bowles, S., & Gintis, H. (2001). The inheritance of economic status: Education, class and genetics. *International Encyclopedia of the Social and Behavioral Sciences: Genetics, Behavior and Society, 6,* 4132–4141.

Chanturidze, G., & Surmava, T. (2021). *The impact of the pandemic on the labor market and the condition of employees*. USAID, East-West Management Institute.

Correia, S., Luck, S., & Verner, E. (2020). *Pandemics depress the economy, public health interventions do not: Evidence from the 1918 flu*. SSRN. https://papers.ssrn.com/sol3/papers.cfm?abstract_id=3561560

Demertzis, M., Sapir, A., Tagliapietra, S., & Wolff, G. B. (2020). An effective economic response to the coronavirus in Europe. *Policy Contributions.*. https://ideas.repec.org/p/bre/polcon/35323.html

Elliot, M. L., & Stephen, M. (2018). *Social mobility: And its enemies*. Penguin.

Elliott, G., Rothenberg, T. J., & Stock, J. H. (1996). Efficient tests for an autoregressive unit root. *Econometrica*, 813–836.

Fairlie, R. W. (2020). The impact of COVID-19 on small business owners: The first three months after social-distancing restrictions. *National Bureau of Economic Research*. https://www.nber.org/papers/w27462

Fasanya, I. O., Oyewole, O., Adekoya, O. B., & Odei-Mensah, J. (2020). Dynamic spillovers and connectedness between COVID-19 pandemic and global foreign exchange markets. *Economic Research-Ekonomska Istrazivanja,* 1–26. https://doi.org/10.1080/1331677X.2020.1860796.

Gangl, M. (2001). European patterns of labour market entry. A dichotomy of occupationalized vs. non-occupationalized systems? *European Societies, 3*(4), 471–494.

Haryanto, T. (2020). Editorial: COVID-19 pandemic and international tourism demand. *Journal of Developing Economies, 5*(1), 1–4.

Ji, X. (2020). A target-oriented bi-attribute user equilibrium model with travelers perception errors on the tolled traffic network. *Transportation Research Part E: Logistics and Transportation Review*. https://doi.org/10.1016/j.tre.2020.102150

Kartseva, M. A., & Kuznetsova, P. O. (2020). The economic consequences of the coronaviru pandemic: Which groups will suffer more in terms of loss of employment and income? *Population and Economics, 4,* 26.

Leka. (2020). An overview of the pandemic impact in the economy of Albania. *The Romanian Economic Journal XXIII, 78,* 2–12.

Ordinance of the Government of Georgia; Retrieved from Legislative Herald of Georgia. (2020, May 23). https://matsne.gov.ge/en/document/view/4877009?publication=161

Lhano, F., & Fonseca, H. (2021). *Covid-19 impact on the labour market of tourism dependent nation (the Southern Europe Case)*. Nova Economics Club.

Li, H., Liu, S. M., Yu, X. H., Tang, S. L., & Tang, C. K. (2020). Coronavirus disease 2019 (COVID-19): Current status and future perspectives. International Journal of Antimicrobial Agents, 55(5), 105951, 2–8. https://doi.org/10.1016/j.ijantimicag.2020.105951.

Lin, P. Z., & Meissner, C. M. (2020). *Health vs. wealth? public health policies and the economy during covid-19*. National Bureau of Economic Research, Inc.

McKibbin, W., & Fernando, R. (2021). The global macroeconomic impacts of COVID-19: Seven scenarios. *Asian Economic Papers, 20*(2), 1–30. Retrieved from https://direct.mit.edu/asep/article-abstract/20/2/1/97314/The-Global-Macroeconomic-Impacts-of-COVID-19-Seven

National Statistics office of Georgia. (2022). Retrieved from National accounts: https://www.geostat.ge/en

Sharma, A., Tiwari, S., Deb, M. K., & Marty, J. L. (2020). Severe acute respiratory syndrome coronavirus-2 (SARS-CoV-2): a global pandemic and treatment strategies. *Journal of Antimicrobial Agents, 56*(2), 106054.

Vanov, D. (2020). Predicting the impacts of epidemic outbreaks on global supply chains: A simulation-based analysis on the coronavirus outbreak (COVID-19/SARS-CoV-2) case Transportation Research Part E. *Logistics and Transportation Review*.

WHO. (2020, January 5). Pneumonia of unknown cause – China. Retrieved November 17,2020, from World Health Organization. https://www.who.int/csr/don/05-january-2020pneumonia-ofunkown-cause-china/en/

Zhang, H., & Shaw, R. (2020). Identifying research trends and gaps in the context of COVID-19. *International Journal of Environmental Research and Public Health, 17*(10). https://doi.org/10.3390/ijerph17103370

Kakhaber-George Lazarashvili   is a Rector of the East European University. Doctor of Education Sciences (UCL, UK). He is a fellow of the Higher Education Academy (UK) and the Member of the Royal Society of Public Health, a Quality Assurance Expert at the University of Greenwich, a Researcher at the UCL-Institute of Education, and a member of the Higher Education Council of the National Center for Educational Quality Enhancement. He is a Senior Lecturer (Healthcare Management). He is a Health and Social Care Management Program Leader at the West London College of Business & Management Sciences, and he holds a Master's Degree in Reproductive Science from the Queen Marry University of London, the author of numerous international scientific articles, a participant of local and international conferences, workshops, seminars, and professional development programmes.

David Sikharulidze   is the Head of the Scientific Research and Development Department of the East European University, an expert of accreditation and authorization of higher education programmes and institutions at the National Center for Educational Quality Enhancement. He has been actively involved in pedagogical and professional activities for many years. He is an invited expert in the field of economics of the Parliament of Georgia, expert in economics of the international organization "International Alert". At various times, he has been studying at the University of Kansas (USA), Metropolitan State University (USA), University of Tartu (Estonia). David is the author and co-author of 4 monographs and 4 textbooks, an author of more than 20 international and local scientific publications, a speaker of up to 20 international and local conferences, a participant of numerous scientific workshops, seminars, an invited expert/evaluator in various international and local grant scientific projects, a participant of up to 30 international professional development events, a participant and researcher of various international and local scientific grant projects.

Tamta Lekishvili   is the Deputy Dean of the Faculty of Business and Engineering at the East European University. She is an Expert in Higher Education at the National Center for Education Quality Enhancement of Georgia. She has been engaged in professional activities for many years. In previous years, she worked in the Quality Assurance Service at the International Black Sea University, held the position of Senior Manager at the Faculty of Business and Engineering at the East European University. Tamta is actively engaged in scientific-research activities. She is the author of up to 10 English-language scientific publications. She has been actively involved in local and international professional development programmes and seasonal schools. Since 2020, Tamta Lekishvili has been a researcher at the Varlam Cherkezishvili Centre for Interdisciplinary Studies at

Eastern European University. At the same time, Tamta Lekishvili is a member of the Dissertation Council of the Eastern European University, Faculty of Business and Engineering.

Vasil Kikutadze is the Dean of the Faculty of Business and Engineering, East European University and the Head of Master's and Bachelor's Programmes in Business Administration. He is an accreditation Expert of Higher Education Programs of the National Center for Educational Quality Enhancement. He has been engaged in professional and pedagogical activities for years in Iv. Javakhishvili Tbilisi State University, Department of Business Organization, Grigol Robakidze University, Parliament's Sector Economy and Economic Policy Committee, Georgian Builders Federation. He has been teaching since 2004. Vasil is the author of one monograph and about 40 scientific local and international publications, a participant and speaker of numerous local and international scientific conferences, seminars, workshops; a supervisor and participant of scientific grant projects. He is actively involved in professional development programmes. He is a member of the editorial board of international scientific peer-reviewed journals.

Chapter 4
What Impact Has the Pandemic Had on the Well-Being of Workers in Germany?

Brigitte Lestrade

Abstract The German authorities' response to the Covid-19 pandemic was slower than elsewhere, due to the country's federal structure, which imposes a division of powers between Berlin and the Länder, with the latter acting in an uncoordinated manner to contain it. It was not until the spring of 2020 that three uniform rules were issued to regulate the behaviour of citizens, while for companies, occupational health and safety rules in a legally binding regulation already applied. Companies, forced to react to the emergency, introduced physical distancing measures on site or allowed employees to work from home, or a combination of both. As a result, the number of teleworkers, which was initially very small, has grown considerably, although not to the extent achieved in other countries.

The numerous surveys conducted by the Ministry of Labour and by independent research institutes to assess the effects of the health situation on work and employment focus mainly on organizational issues, and studies analysing the development of the sense of well-being of German employees are only marginally included. However, the questionnaires submitted to them show that the mental state of employees does not seem to have been significantly affected by the reorganization of the pandemic, with women being slightly less optimistic than men, and employees working from home even less so than those who had stayed at home. Overall, employees are satisfied with the way their employer has handled the health situation, often without the coaching of consulting firms, which are not very common in Germany.

The Covid-19 pandemic poses a new challenge for companies and their employees in terms of the speed with which these economic actors have had to deal with this new situation and the need to learn from it for the future. It is essential to study the new challenges for both companies and their employees. Companies are facing loss

Translated from French to English by Louise Dalingwater.

B. Lestrade (✉)
University of Cergy-Pontoise, Cergy-Pontoise, France

of revenue, financial uncertainty, and disruption of supply chains, not to mention the need for contingency plans in the event of economic disruption. How companies, large and small, cope with this turmoil depends on a variety of factors. If a company is to survive in today's ever-changing and challenging environment, it must consider both the physical and mental well-being, of its critically important employees, who are difficult to replace in the short term.

The pandemic has not only disrupted normal business life, it has also had a major impact on the mental well-being of every employee, not only those who are ultimately risking their lives as health care workers, but also those for whom working from home can be a daily experience of isolation. As stress levels increase, it becomes more difficult for employees to focus on their work. This makes it all the more important for employers to know what their employees are facing, both at home and in the workplace, so that they can best support them in the new situation.

The first part of this study, which focuses on the impact of the pandemic on the well-being of employees in Germany (the inequality aspect is largely absent for structural reasons, as will be discussed later), outlines the regulatory framework, which is all the more necessary as Germany, as a federal state, must constantly navigate between the competences of Berlin and the significant powers granted to the governments of the *Länder*. Then we will study the measures put in place by companies to protect their employees as best they can while limiting the negative impact on their activities. As the German government has imposed the use of remote working wherever possible, the measures taken by companies to comply with it will be discussed, as well as the consequences of these changes on employees, both from an organizational point of view and in terms of their impact on their mental state. Most of them are convinced that reorganizations implemented by companies will continue after the end of the pandemic.

4.1   Health Rules to Follow in the Event of a Pandemic

The concrete impact of a pandemic, such as Covid-19, on the lives of a country's citizens stems from two packages of measures, the one that the state imposes on all its inhabitants and the one that applies to companies. As Germany is a federal state, most of the provisions that regulate life in society come from the governments of the 16 *Länder* that make up the country, from the smallest, Bremen, with its 680,000 inhabitants, to the most populous, North Rhine-Westphalia, with almost 18 million inhabitants. This division of powers, jealously guarded by regional officials, meant that the Berlin government took a long time, more than a year, before it succeeded in imposing a set of rules (on 22 March 2021, called the "emergency brake"

(Notbremse), which applied uniformly throughout the country from an incidence rate of more than 100.[1]

4.1.1   National Rules that Apply to All Germans

These rules, only three in total because the state administrations have not been able to agree on greater convergence, are as follows:

- Private contact: a household may meet at most one other person.
- Curfew in case of high incidence:[2] from 10 p.m. to 5 a.m., possibility to play sports until midnight.
- Schools: testing twice a week with alternating classes. With an incidence of more than 165 on 3 consecutive days, all classes will be taught remotely at home.

While the rules governing the behaviour of citizens may vary from state to state, apart from these three national rules decided by the Berlin government, the rules governing the operation of companies with regard to employee protection are those that apply to all companies in Germany, regardless of their size or field of activity. The occupational health and safety regulations, supplemented by the specific provisions for combating Covid-19, are part of a comprehensive system of occupational health and safety regulations.

4.1.2   Rules That Apply to All Companies

- Strict compliance to the minimum distance of 1.5 m between two persons; wearing of mouth and nose protection (medical masks), where this cannot be observed and where the installation of movable partitions is not possible.
- Compliance with the minimum distance of 1.5 m also in canteens and rest rooms.
- Provision of liquid soap and towel dispensers in toilets.
- Regular and adequate ventilation.

---

[1] If an incidence of 100 cases is exceeded in a county or non-county city for 3 consecutive days, the nationwide emergency brake will automatically be applied there beginning the next day. For incidences below 100, each state continues to decide what rules and restrictions to apply. The guidelines for this are determined jointly by the federal government and the *Länder*. In addition, each *Land* can also go beyond the emergency brake with its own measures in the case of impacts above 100.

[2] The curfew introduced with the "federal emergency brake" between 10 p.m. and 5 a.m. in districts and cities with a high 7-day incidence had little effect on the night time mobility of the population in Germany, according to Destatis, the Federal Statistics Agency: in the period from 24 April to 1 May 2021, night time mobility in counties where a curfew was in effect decreased by only 12% compared to counties without a curfew (PRESSEMITTEILUNG des Statistischen Bundesamtes (DESTATIS) Nr. 215 of 06.05.2021).

- If the same workplace is used by several people, provide 10 m^2 per person.
- In companies with 10 or more employees, division into fixed working groups which should be as small as possible
- Obligation for the employer to provide at the very least medical masks (mouth-nose protection).
- Obligation for the employer to offer a corona test at least twice a week to all employees who do not work exclusively from home.
- Use of appropriate telecommunication means for meetings.
- Flexible working: the former provisions of the Corona Ordinance on Occupational Health and Safety concerning home offices have been transferred to the Infection Protection Act and made more restrictive.[3] Employers are therefore still required to offer the possibility to work from home, unless there are compelling operational reasons not to. Employees are also required to accept these offers, unless there are compelling reasons to refuse.

The occupational health and safety rules in the Covid-19 Pandemic Occupational Health and Safety Ordinance have been supplemented with new provisions on the frequency of testing, increasing to at least two tests per week to be offered to employees as of 23 April. The period of validity of the rules applicable in companies is planned to run until 30 June 2021 inclusive, with all previous provisions of the ordinance remaining unchanged. The application of the Covid-19 occupational health and safety regulations comes with a presumption of compliance, i.e. if the measures described therein are complied with, the employer can assume that the occupational health and safety requirements are met. However, the employer is free to take other measures if they are equally effective in safeguarding the physical and mental health and well-being of his employees.

Display in German companies:

---

[3] Occupational Protection Ordinance SARS-CoV-2(Corona-ArbSchV):

Controlling SARS-CoV-2 and preventing its spread requires effective and coordinated measures to avoid contact with people and to provide sufficient protection against infection in all areas of life, i.e., in private life, society, and the workplace.

Since in many areas of life the possibilities for further limiting contact and for additional infection protection measures are largely exhausted, additional and temporary occupational protection measures in the workplace are indispensable to contribute to the protection of workers' health.

The Corona-ArbSchV ordinance and its basic occupational health and safety regulations are extended until 19 March 2022.

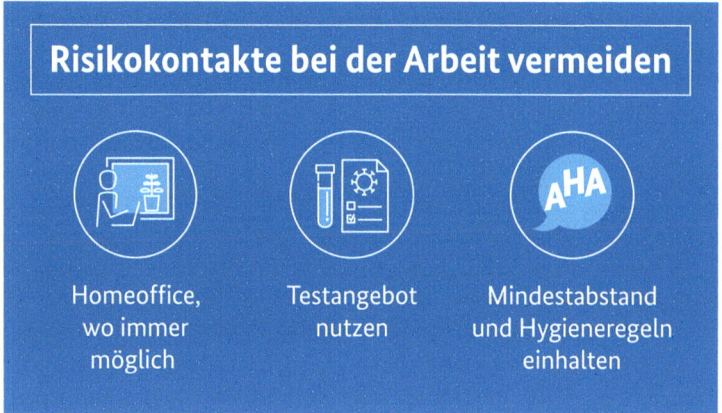

Text: Work from home wherever possible, take advantage of the test offer, comply with the rules on minimum distancing and hygiene rules (Application planned by the government until 20.3.2022).

4.2   The Reaction of Companies to the Restrictions Imposed by the Public Authorities

Compelled to respect the legal constraints imposed by the public authorities in order to limit the spread of the virus, companies which were anxious to keep their businesses going as best they could, had to either keep their employees on site by adapting their premises to respect the distancing instructions, or propose remote work, or even a combination of both. Aware of the impact that this new situation could have on the physical and mental health of their employees, companies took action in two directions, namely, the introduction of remote working where feasible to reduce the risk of contamination, and the use of psychological support methods to help their staff cope with the disruption to their daily lives.

4.3   Moderate Increase in Remote Working

In contrast to other European countries, notably France and Belgium, where remote working was mandatory wherever feasible, in Germany the government's rules on remote working were initially interpreted by both companies and employees as recommendations rather than injunctions. It was not until 27 January 2021 that the German government, in agreement with the *Länder*, decided to make remote working in companies mandatory. This Homeoffice-Pflicht specifies that the employer is obliged to offer his or her employees the possibility of working from home, as long as there are no business-related reasons against it. Employees, on the other hand, are free to accept or refuse this offer. Many activities, particularly in industry and construction, do not lend themselves to a move to working from home, but where this was possible, employers were obliged to offer remote working to their employees, an offer more easily accepted by people with a high level of education and income.

Remote working has developed in a variable way, rather modest overall, depending on the evolution of the pandemic, on the one hand, and the legal environment on the other. From only 4% before the start of the pandemic, the rate of employees working from home increased to 27% during the first lockdown in the early fall of 2020,[4] and then dropped to 14% in November 2020. In February 2021, following the government's decision to make remote working compulsory wherever practicable, around 30% of employees were working from home, either partially or completely, a figure which is well below the potential, which has been estimated at 56% (Alipour et al., 2021, ifo).

This reluctance, which is mainly due to the fear of an unknown illness that could affect their physical health and well-being, is due to the employees rather than the companies, as the share of those who offer remote working to their employees stood at 81% in February 2021. However, the possibility offered by some companies does not seem to have convinced their employees, as the acceptance rate is very different depending on the field of activity. The service sector has the largest share of remote workers, standing at 40%. In the wholesale trade, the figure is 24%, in industry just under 22% (Alipour, ifo-Schnelldienst, 6/2021). All studies show that small- and medium-sized companies have converted to telework much less than large companies. However, even before the current Covid-19 pandemic, working from home was much more common in large companies than in small- or medium-sized ones. This reluctance is considered unfortunate in the current situation by both governments and research institutes, because all surveys have shown that remote working is an effective lever against the pandemic because, as reported in the Ifo Institute survey cited above, employees who work face to face are four to eight times more likely to report a Covid-19 infection than those who work from home.

According to a study conducted by the Ministry of Labour and Social Affairs (Bonin et al., 2021), which analyses the attitudes of German employees towards remote working, the new, more stringent regulations have indeed had an impact on their behaviour in this respect. In the survey, one in four employees stated that this new provision has changed the use of home-office work in their own company. Many employees who expressed this view noted that co-workers who did not previously work from home have begun to do so, and that co-workers who previously worked from home have increased the amount of time spent in the home office. Employees who have not seen a change in the practice of remote working at their company as a result of the government's HHS Ordinance cite two main reasons: first,

---

[4]The dates varied according to the Länder, which had very important powers granted by the government in Berlin.

	Sector	Total	SME/SMI	Large companies
Table 4.1 Remote working in February 2021, by sector and company size	Total economy	30.3	26.1	39.3
	Industry	21.5	15.3	31.1
	Total services	40.9	37.8	49.5
	Total trade	18.2	13.1	28.9
	Wholesale trade	24.3	19.1	31.2
	Retail trade	9.8	7.3	21.4
	Total construction	10.1	6.1	19.4

Source: ifo Konjunkturumfrage, February 2021, published in ifo-Schnelldienst 6/2021

remote working was already possible for individuals at their company before, and second, the work performed at their company does not lend itself well to this practice (Table 4.1).

The fact, also observed in earlier studies, that the activities of many employees are not really suitable for remote working, seems to be the most important factor for respondents to explain why remote working has not been used more in the current health situation. In contrast, only about one in five employees cited the lack or poor quality of technical equipment as the main reason for the absence or inadequacy of flexible working in their establishment. Therefore, the Occupational Health and Safety Ordinance is likely to impact on the behaviour of employees who already perform their work at least partially from home. Of these, one in four employees said they would ask their employer to increase the portion of their business which is conducted from home for this reason.

However, a large majority of employees surveyed were satisfied with the current amount of work done at home or consider that they already do as much as the nature of their work allows. Of those employees who do not currently work from home, one in ten reported that they were considering asking their employer to allow them to do so, citing the ordinance as the reason for their request. In very few cases, this reluctance was justified by the fear that such a request might be perceived badly by the employer.

While flexible working has increased since the outbreak of the pandemic, it is essentially as a result of the fear, on the part of both employers and employees, of its impact on the physical well-being of the latter. What is missing from the debate in Germany, however, is the inequality aspect that seems to exist in other European countries where relations within companies are regulated differently. The main reason for the harmonious relations within companies is a certain equality of powers between managers and employees, introduced in particular by the law on co-determination (Gesetz über die Mitbestimmung der Arbeitnehmer vom 4.5.1976 (BGBl. I 1153)). This created a quasi-parity in the supervisory board in companies with more than 2000 employees, which ensures that decisions are taken by all parties concerned.[5] If the *Mitbestimmung* intended by the legislator allows for harmonious social relations within large companies, the existence of the *Betriebsräte*,[6] work councils which regulate social relations in all companies with 5 or more employees, does not guarantee an absence of conflict, but the resolution of conflict in the interest of all parties. The very broad powers of German employees not only allow them to make their voices heard by their superiors on any subject that concerns them, they also give them the means to ensure that all members of their community are treated equally. This is why the question of inequalities within companies, whether in the context of the pandemic or otherwise, does not arise in Germany. On the other hand, the differences in regulations in the different *Länder*—whether schools are closed or not, access to restaurants, etc.—are perceived very differently in Germany. But these inequalities are not a matter for the German government but the responsibility of companies.

4.4   The Impact of Remote Working on Employees' Family Activities

While companies are obliged to find organizational and technical solutions for the introduction of remote working, employees have to deal with the constraints that come with the cohabitation of family and professional activities. In addition to the need to find a location where they can concentrate on their work, many employees are also faced with the challenge of reconciling their work and family activities, including the supervision of children at home, which is very common in the context of the pandemic. Germany's national regulation, the Notbremse is very specific on this subject: if the incidence level exceeds 100 cases for 3 consecutive days, all schools are required to alternate between face-to-face and distance learning. In concrete terms, by the end of April 2021, almost half of the municipalities exceeded the incidence of 165 cases, which meant in practice that 11 million children under the age of 14 were out of school and that about a quarter of German employees had a childcare problem.

---

[5] In order to avoid a deadlock in the decision-making process between representatives of the capital and the employees, the chairman of the supervisory board has a double vote to decide on controversial issues. The use of this possibility is extremely rare, as the two sides of industry in Germany always tend to reach a consensus.

[6] Seventy years ago, on 14 November 1952, the *Betriebsverfassungsgesetz* (Works Constitution Act) came into force. In the tradition of the Weimar Works Council Act, it regulates the extensive information, consultation, and co-determination rights of the works council and prescribes a "trust-based cooperation" between the company management and the work council. Work councils are elected in workplaces with at least five permanent employees who are entitled to vote, of whom three are eligible. These elections are held every 4 years, usually in May. The most recent elections took place between May 1 and 31, 2022.

4.5   No Rebalancing of Tasks in the Home

As a result of the economic downturn in Germany, with the closure of many stores and the reduction in the production of non-essential goods, many employees have been or are being forced to reduce or stop work altogether in order to care for their children, with the closure of day care centres and schools. This combination of reduced employment, on the one hand, and increased childcare on the other, has had a significant impact on the distribution of family work within the household. The new possibilities of reconciliation through flexible work at home should make it possible to better reconcile work and domestic tasks and to distribute the care of the couple's children more equally among the caregivers.

However, a survey conducted by the WSI Institute (Kohlrausch & Zucco, 2020) clearly shows that, even in times of crisis, the overwhelming majority of work in the household and childcare is done by women. 54% of the women surveyed, but only 12% of the men, said that they take on the majority of childcare tasks. This is consistent with existing patterns of gendered division of labour, as childcare was also largely performed by women before the pandemic. Only one-third of respondents reported that childcare is shared equally by both parents. This assessment is expressed equally by men and women. Only in a small proportion of couples do men assume the majority of child care. Thus, the proportion of men assuming the largest share increased from 6 to 12% during the pandemic.[7]

While men's involvement in family tasks is far from equal to that of women, there are still differences in this area between women in the East and West of what was the Wall during the GDR. Before unification, East German women were all employed outside the home due to political pressure, whereas in the West, if women had jobs at all, they were mostly part-time, as childcare facilities were very limited. Since unification, childcare outside the home has changed significantly in both East and West Germany. These changes resulted not only from the systemic upheaval, which led to a reorganization of the content and structure of the childcare system in East Germany, but also from the growing need of West German parents for full-time childcare facilities. This growing demand was mainly due to the increase in women's employment and the resulting expectations regarding the reconciliation of work and family life. The fact that the majority of East German women have considered, and still consider, it natural to work alongside their desire to have children, and the economic independence this brings, has led to changes in the attitudes of West German men and women towards women's work and the reconciliation of family and work life. The inequalities that may have existed during the period when Germany was divided into two politically, economically, and socially separate states are disappearing: the employment rate of women in the West is close to that of

---

[7]This increase in men's participation in household activities and childcare is likely to have a long-term impact. It has been shown (Tamm, 2019) that even a few months of parental leave, and thus time during which fathers take on childcare, has long-term effects on a more egalitarian division of domestic labour.

women in the East, even if, because of the childcare facilities that often continue to operate only in the morning, they work part-time more often than their counterparts in the East. In this respect, it is the behaviour of women in the East that has rubbed off on that of women in the West. The data on this subject do not take into account whether attitudes have remained the same or changed since the onset of the pandemic.

A study by the Federal Ministry of Labour and Social Affairs (Bonin et al., 2021) also showed that women are less well equipped by their employers with the equipment they need to perform their duties at home, such as a laptop, desktop computer, or even an office chair: while only 6% of male employees did not receive any work-related equipment from their employer, the figure for women is 11%, a discrepancy that cannot be explained by the nature of the work to be performed. Unfortunately, the study did not provide any information that could explain this discrepancy.

4.6 Employees' Nuanced Assessment of the Impact of the Remote Working Systems in Place

From an employee perspective, employers are doing well overall in their efforts to protect against infection, according to a governmental study (Bonin et al., 2021). Only 17% are currently very or extremely concerned that they could be infected with coronavirus at work. Only one in ten employees feel that their employer's measures to protect them from infection are not sufficiently thorough on the whole. On the other hand, 82% of employees consider the measures taken by their employer to protect them from infection to be quite adequate. Their assessment of the impact of the home office on their mental state is also fairly positive.

A representative study conducted from 23 November 2020 to 11 December 2020 by the psyga.info Institute[8] provided detailed results on employees' perceptions of the effects of remote working on their well-being. The statements to be commented on were:

• My performance whilst working from home compared to working in the office is higher
  than usual ($n = 1601$ at least one day per week of remote working).

---

[8]PsyGa's sample of respondents included 4970 employees, including 1379 management personnel and 3591 non-management personnel; 32% worked from home at least one day per week, 12% were partially unemployed. The survey was conducted in two stages, once during the week after Easter 2020, in the middle of the first lockdown, and in late November and early December 2020. The results discussed above are from the second wave of the study. PsyGA (Psychische Gesundheit in der Arbeitswelt), which is part of the Institut Neue Qualität der Arbeit (INQA), is supported by the Federal Ministry of Labor and Social Affairs. (https://www.psyga.info/corona-umfrage#:~: text=Hier%20sind%20die%20wichtigsten%20Ergebnisse. & text=Jede%20siebte%20Person% 2C%20d.h.%2014.5,psychisch%20relevant%20besser%20als%202019).

- I feel very well informed by my employer about how we should act in this situation.
- The support of my employer in this situation is exemplary.
- My employer is working to fight the pandemic even outside and beyond the company.
- The situation has strengthened the feeling of belonging to our working group.
- I have finally managed to do some nice things that I wouldn't have time for otherwise.

  The employees surveyed (for their socio-economic level, see note 4 in Chap. 2) had a choice of five responses ranging from total agreement to total disagreement. The briefly summarized results of the survey, compared to those conducted previously, are as follows:
- On average, the employees surveyed are psychologically stable. Those who participated in all three surveys show on average a slight deterioration in their well-being.
- One in seven respondents, or 14.5%, reported a significant deterioration in their mental well-being.
- One in eleven, or 9.1%, consider themselves to be in a better psychological situation than in 2019. The evaluation of one's own performance when working from home has increased compared to the March statements.
- The perceived impact on the "feeling of belonging to the group" has decreased compared to March.
- The assessment of the need to work more than usual has increased again compared to
  March.
- Two-thirds of employees consider their employer to be supportive in an exemplary manner, unchanged from the first lockdown.

Many of the studies that have been conducted on the impact of remote working on the lives of employees essentially point to the increased pressure from companies to finish the work they have started, which leads to frequent overtime. In addition, there is a certain amount of mental fatigue that is no longer counterbalanced by physical fatigue, particularly because of the elimination of the walk to work. The lack of social contact is also often mentioned, especially the elimination of informal breaks in the workplace, which used to help not only to decompress, but also to convey professional or non-professional information that served as a link between colleagues. The impossible task of clearly separating private time from work time is also cited negatively in most studies on this topic.

However, most studies conclude that it is not the work from home itself that causes the mental and emotional exhaustion cited by many employees. According to the University of Konstanz study (Kunze et al., 2021), 26% of respondents working from home reported feeling emotionally exhausted and drained, whereas only 21% of employees working from home did so. Without analysing this difference in perception, the authors of the study point out that the majority of respondents do not want to return to compulsory full-time presence in the company: 56% of them want to be able to work at least partially from home. For many respondents, the desired model is a balanced mix of working from home and being present in the company. While 25% of respondents want to work entirely remotely, the majority of them prefer 2–3 days a week of working from home (average of all respondents: 2.88 days). 50% of them are in favour of a right to remote working (Kunze et al., 2021).

4.7   What Initiatives have Companies Taken to Support the Well-Being of Their Employees?

The fact that remote workers are slightly less mentally exhausted than those who go to the office every day shows that this choice by the government and companies was appropriate in the present situation. Nevertheless, a small or large quarter of employees, depending on whether they work at home or at the office, suffer emotionally. Most studies from official sources or research institutes focus on organizational and performance issues of employees, whether they work from home or not. Well-being is very rarely mentioned, sometimes for those who work remotely, but almost never about employees who continue to travel to their work-place. These are mainly those whose professional activity cannot be carried out remotely, i.e. manual activities, in factories or stores, for example, whose staff are particularly exposed to the risks inherent in the pandemic. However, the latter are equally, if not more, affected by the health situation and its constraints. Since the public authorities have enacted rules on the protection of the physical health of employees only, it was therefore up to the companies themselves to ensure the mental well-being of their staff.

However, most of them, especially SMEs, are not prepared to set up a protocol likely to prevent or treat the ill-being of their employees, whether they work on site or remotely. There is also an offer from some consulting firms that provide services to guide management personnel in their tasks of reassuring and comforting their staff in this unknown and worrying environment. However, unlike in other countries, especially in the Anglosphere, they are not very common. To date, no study on the impact of consulting firms in managing employee well-being has been published.[9] However, some of them, especially those that focus on the physical health of employees in the workplace, have developed rules that can be adopted to support their mental well-being in the current health situation.

Many employees not only suffer from the disruption of their work routines and contact restrictions, they also worry about the possibility of partial or frictional unemployment, the risk of their company going bankrupt, the uncertain future, an anxiety-provoking situation reinforced by the media and social networks. Some consulting

---

[9]On the other hand, there are more than seven million technical notes on the Internet about employee well-being in German companies.

firms offer companies coaching measures to improve the well-being of their employees in this stressful situation.

A synthesis of their recommendations as well as those of the German Ministry of Labour and the German health insurance companies offers companies a common thread that can facilitate personnel management that takes into account the constraints imposed by the pandemic. Most of the tips for improving employee well-being in the anxiety-arousing context of the pandemic suggest the following approaches:

- **Support employees who work from home:**

  – Make management aware of their employees' need for moral support
  – Create a communication plan to regularly inform employees of new information and regulations to create transparency
  – Increase the number of video conferences, both for business and non-business purposes
  – Provide more flexibility for employees to better balance work and family activities

- **Improve existing programmes:**

  – Increase access to company-sponsored health programmes
  – Provide or improve information about employee and family well-being
  – Supplement existing programmes with coaching sessions if necessary

- **Reduce stress and anxiety**:

  – Offer seminars on resilience and stress management
  – Increase access to online fitness sessions
  – Target particularly vulnerable groups of employees
  – Create opportunities for virtual meetings after work

While much of the advice given to companies on how to manage the disruption of the pandemic and its impact on employees' mental health has come from organizations eager to sell their expertise, most managers and their employees have shown that they are able to cope with the upheaval of their internal organization and adapt to the circumstances. While everyone wants to return to a state free from the constraints of the health situation imposed by Covid-19, it is clear to most employees and their management that a return to pre-pandemic organizational structures is not an option.

4.8   What Impact Will the Pandemic Have on Work Organization in the Future?

Prior to the pandemic, remote working in Germany was low by international standards. The mandatory employee protection regulations issued by Berlin and state governments led to a massive increase in teleworking, a new experience for many employees. While the return to the office after the crisis is likely to be welcomed by many, it is a fact that this legislative environment now allows employers to introduce flexible working if it is necessary for health reasons, especially since teleworkers have shown that they are as productive working from home as they are on their employer's premises, or even more so according to some expert reports (Rief, 2021).

This change in the work environment, described as hybrid between face-to-face and remote work, has led the government to consider the possibility of introducing a right to telework for employees. The Federal Ministry of Labour has considered the possibility of introducing a right to work from home, according to which all employees whose work can be done at home would have the right to freely choose their place of work for a certain number of days per year. However, these plans were overwhelmingly rejected by the German population. A majority (56%) are not in favour of a legal right to telework, as currently under discussion. Of those surveyed, 40% welcomed the Ministry's proposal. This is the result of a representative survey of more than 1000 people aged 16 and over in Germany, commissioned by the digital association Bitkom in late October 2020. This is an issue which divides generations: while the majority of 16–29 year olds (51%) welcome the plan, 58% of those aged 30 and over oppose it.

While many employees have a positive experience of remote working, more positive than initially assumed, a majority of them are critical of the proposed legal right to work from home. This is because, according to Bitkom researchers, they fear that such legislation could lead to a two-tier society among employees. For almost half of the respondents (48%), the argument against the right to work from home was the injustice done to colleagues whose work is not suitable for remote work. Among those opposed to the right to work from home, 63%, cite this reason. 40% of respondents feared having less contact and exchange with their colleagues and 53% of those who were opposed to remote working. Just over one-third of respondents (32%) believed that their colleagues working from home would work less; this figure is higher (45%) among those who oppose it. And one in five (20%) saw it as an unacceptable encroachment on entrepreneurial freedom and one in three (32%) of those who oppose remote working shared this view. One in six (17%) was concerned about data security and one in five (20%) of those opposed to the remote working bill.

The findings of the various employee surveys show that employees are convinced that the organization of work should not be imposed by the state, but should be defined within the company between employers and employees. They believe that modern forms of flexible working are not an end in themselves and must be in harmony with the corporate culture and integrated into the internal processes of the company. With this in mind, the Bitkom researchers who analysed the data recommend that the state should provide incentives for flexible working time and place, without over-regulating in this area. They also believe that those who regularly work from home should be put on an equal footing with commuters in terms of taxation, as they avoid traffic congestion and protect the environment. The same goes for remote workers' investment in computer equipment: they too should receive a one-time tax bonus. Some researchers go even further and advocate that in the long term the equipment of all employees likely to do home-office work should be supported, either by the state or by the employer, or both.

4.9   Conclusion

The response to the outbreak of the pandemic in Germany was late, both on the part of the government and the business community. The federal structure of the country, which allows for a great deal of latitude for decision-making to the *Länder*, led to a delayed response from the central government in Berlin, which just issued a few general health rules. From the end of 2019 until the spring of 2020, companies were in a relative limbo, with the measures taken by the *Länder* varying greatly from one Land to another. Companies have introduced distance measures in their premises and instructed employees whose activity lends itself to it and who consent to it to work from home. Compared to other European countries, Germany normally has a relatively low rate of remote working. The majority of those who are allowed to work from home prefer to work in the office, as several surveys have shown. The main reasons for this are the need for direct personal interaction in the office and the fact that people consider that their own way of working requires personal presence.

In view of the late but energetic reaction of companies that have considerably expanded access to the home office, leading to a significant increase in the number of teleworkers, some research institutes have investigated the consequences of these changes on the well-being of workers suddenly confronted with a major change in their working environment. The results of the surveys showed that employees were aware of the effect of these changes in their working environment on their well-being, both in a positive and negative sense.

In many cases, the negative emphasis is on the fact that this form of work leads to difficulties to separate work and private life. This statement comes from employees who work from home as well as from those who are mainly in the office within the company. These interferences can lead to significant psychological stress. Rest periods are reduced or can no longer be clearly defined, especially when working from home in the evening or at weekends. However, the negative impact of the health constraints due to the pandemic is hardly perceptible through the surveys, perhaps because German companies have been able to support their employees during these transformations of their working environment. This finding is supported by the fact that many employees who were not familiar with remote working say they are ready to adopt it, even without health restrictions.

The majority of respondents to various surveys are convinced that location-independent working will increase. For example, more than half of them expect the proportion of employees who work fully or partially from home to increase over the next 5 years, perhaps because some of them have discovered, and some surveys have confirmed, that working from home can also have a beneficial impact on their well-being.

References

Alipour, J. V., Falck, O., Peichel, A. Sauer, S. (2021). *Homeoffice-Potenziel weiterhin nicht ausgeschöpft, ifo-Schnelldienst 6/2021.*

Bonin, H., Krause-Pilatus, A., Rinne, U.. (2021). *Arbeitssituation und Belastungsempfinden im Kontext der Corona-Pandemie, IZA-Kurzexpertise im Auftrag des Bundesministeriums für Arbeit und Soziales.* http://ftp.iza.org/report_pdfs/iza_report_117.pdf

Kohlrausch, B., & Zucco, A. (2020 May). *Die Corona-Krise trifft Frauen doppelt, Wirtschafts- und Sozialwissenschaftliches Institut (WSI) der Hans-Böckler-Stiftung, Nr. 40.*

Kunze F., Hampel, K., & Zimmermann, S. (2021, July 16). *Homeoffice in der Corona-Krise: eine nachhaltige Transformation der Arbeitswelt?* Policy Paper N° 02, Universität Konstanz, Homeoffice in der Corona-Krise: eine nachhaltige Transformation der Arbeitswelt? (uni-konstanz.de).

Rief, S. (2021). *Dr.: Auf dem Weg in eine hybride Arbeitswelt – Büros und Büroarbeit in der Post-Corona-Epoche.* https://forum.dguv.de/ausgabe/3-2021/artikel/auf-dem-weg-in-eine-hybride-arbeitswelt-bueros-und-bueroarbeit-in-der-post-corona-epoche

Tamm, M. (2019). Fathers' parental leave-taking, childcare involvement and labor market participation. *Labour Economics, 59,* 184–197.

Brigitte Lestrade is Emeritus Professor of contemporary German studies at the University of Cergy-Pontoise and member of the editorial board of the journal *Allemagne Aujourd'hui*. She also gives lectures at Paris Nanterre and at the Ecole Polytechnique, the Université du Littoral. She was previously the director of a department, faculty dean, vice-president of the board of directors in charge of international affairs and communication at Dunkirk, then vice-president in charge of international affairs at Cergy. She has written many articles and books on the economic, sociological and cultural aspects of Germany today, especially on the world of work.

Chapter 5
Covid-19 and Well-Being Policies in Ireland. A Preliminary Study with a Focus on Young People

Vanessa Boullet and Julien Guillaumond

Abstract In April 2020, the Central Statistics Office (CSO) released the results of its Social Impact of Covid-19 survey on well-being in the Republic of Ireland. Since then, some further results were published in August and November 2020, and February 2021, offering a year-long review on well-being in Ireland during the pandemic. In February 2021, as Ireland experienced the "most stringent lockdown" among European nations, Irish people's well-being indicators worsened, even though a series of measures had been implemented by the Irish State to alleviate the economic and social consequences of Covid-19 on the population, and Irish businesses.

Interestingly, the Irish coalition led by Micheál Martin (Fianna Fáil) placed the notion of well-being at the core of its strategy. The Programme for Government: Our shared future, published in June 2020, stated: "The well-being of our nation, however, goes beyond the narrow confines of economic growth. Over the next 5 years, the Government will use well-being indicators as well as economic indicators to point out inequalities and help ensure that policies are driven by a desire to do better by people" [4].

A series of questions form the core of this chapter: Has the definition of well-being in Ireland been transformed by the Covid-19 pandemic? Are well-being indicators under consideration by the Irish State addressing the needs of specific

---

This chapter is part of ongoing research by the two authors on the economic and social consequences of Covid-19 on Irish society. As it is a real-time study, its results will only be tentative since Ireland was still in the midst of the pandemic at the time of writing (May 2022), and the full impact of the pandemic has not been fully assessed, be it in Ireland or in any other countries.

V. Boullet (✉)
Université de Lorraine, Nancy, France
e-mail: vanessa.boullet@univ-lorraine.fr

J. Guillaumond
Université Clermont Auvergne, Clermont Auvergne, France
e-mail: julien.guillaumond@uca.fr

people? Would the implementation of economic and social measures mark a shift towards a fairer and happier Irish society?

5.1 Introduction

On 11 March 2020, the World Health Organization stated that Covid-19/Sars-Cov2 had reached pandemic status (World Health Organization, 2020). Throughout the world, Governments had already started to fight against this new disease, and this new step drove many countries to launch emergency responses to protect both their populations and their economies, setting up crisis response teams to oversee state's reactions (quest for face masks and later, vaccine), and also designing and implementing economic and social measures to alleviate the impacts of Covid-19 and its forced lockdowns on economic activity (such as various grants and tax reliefs or exemptions) and on people's standards of living to compensate for the loss of income. Retrospectively, within OECD countries, one could say that well-being in its broader sense was again emphasized since governments did their utmost to protect their citizens and care for them through various national efforts, suggesting that the welfare state was still relevant. Such a point was recalled by the Irish Minister for Social Protection, Heather Humphreys, when she stated that Covid-19 had shown the importance of providing a safety net for all citizens (Economic & Social Research Institute, 2021).

After the initial shock of discovering that pandemics had not disappeared, that Covid-19 could well turn out to be similar to the great Spanish flu of the early twentieth century, and looking at rising mortality rates which caused much concern for people's lives and well-being, the next step was to react and adapt to that unexpected situation. As the WHO Director-General said, the world "[had] never before seen a pandemic sparked by a coronavirus. This is the first pandemic caused by a coronavirus. And we have never before seen a pandemic that can be controlled, at the same time" (World Health Organization, 2020). And yet, control quickly took various forms, mostly gradual restrictions of liberties and lockdowns, while questions arose as to the origins of such a virus and its effects on people. Though lockdowns had some severe impacts on economic activity, research continued on Covid-19 to find some vaccines (and on its successive variants as the world was soon to discover) as well as on ways to prepare for an uncertain future (for example, on strategies to release lockdowns) while trying to assess the current economic, social, and political consequences of the pandemic on societies and people's lives as time went by.

5.2   Covid-19 and Well-Being Research

Well-being and the impacts of the pandemic on mental health became the focus of much research. The Covid-19 pandemic has become, for some, "a prime example for the economic study of subjective well-being, with the ultimate purpose of comprehensively assessing the welfare consequences of the pandemic and associated policy measures" (Schmidtke et al., 2021). In other words, it has become a new focus of real-time study with the definition of new approaches on well-being, and its inclusion in new policy formulation in the future. Such a perspective still contains some limitations. Indeed, as research often feeds itself from previous data and experience, and as the world had not known such a situation on this scale in the past, there was always a degree of uncertainty, and the idea that research was in the making was truly meaningful. To date, most research has not provided any definite answer and in terms of well-being, there are more long-term implications on individuals' lives and behaviours which are not yet studied and/or known.

Successive studies attest to the negative impacts of Covid on well-being. It has been found that the different policies states implemented following the outbreak of the disease (physical distancing and various social restrictions), together with Covid-19 itself, had some true negative impacts on mental health (Banks et al., 2021). Various "stressors" linked to health consequences (infection/death), financial consequences (unemployment, *etc.*), daily life consequences (domestic arrangements, family settings), and loss of freedom and activity, leading to social disconnection and isolation are truly revealing regarding the impact of the pandemic on people's lives (Banks et al., 2021). Covid also had an impact on psychological well-being across the world, and consequently, happiness and life satisfaction declined (Okabe-Miyamoto & Lyubomrisky, 2021). Finally, international studies reveal that Covid had an impact on workers' well-being. Though different economic sectors dealt with its consequences differently, it triggered further inequalities in the world of work,[1] leading to a shift to telework, and possible changes to the future of work. In Germany, for instance, it has been found that the pandemic had negative effects on mental health and on life satisfaction of workers, though between the waves, there was some return to normality through adaptation (Schmidtke et al., 2021). Until recently, it appears that the definition of well-being has been rarely discussed in academic work in Ireland.[2] And at the time of writing [May 2022], there are very few studies which have formally questioned the Covid pandemic and its positive or

---

[1] See, for instance, Maria Cotofan, Jan-Emmanuel De Neve, Marta Golin, Micah Kaats, George Ward, "Work and Well-being during Covid-19: Impact, Inequalities, Resilience, and the Future of Work", *in* John F. Helliwell, Richard Layard, Jeffrey D. Sachs, Jan-Emmanuel De Neve, Lara B. Aknin, and Shun Wang, *World Happiness Report 2021*, pp. 153–190.

[2] In Ireland, research often tends to associate well-being with happiness or life satisfaction. For example, David Madden in "The Impact of an Economic Boom on the Level and Distribution of Well-Being: Ireland, 1994–2001" (2010) or Brendan M. Walsh in "Well-being and economic conditions in Ireland" (2011) discuss subjective well-being as being close to happiness and life satisfaction.

negative consequences on well-being in Ireland, except for research of the Economic and Social Research Institute (ESRI). In an article for the *Irish Medical Journal* late 2020, B. D. Kelly was convinced that the Covid-19 pandemic would have effects on the mental health of the general population in Ireland as elsewhere (Kelly, 2020).[3] Those effects would of course be more acute among people with mental illnesses, but also among the general population because of increased anxiety and the effects of imposed restrictions on people.

5.3   The Outbreak of Covid-19 in Ireland and the State's Response

On 29 February 2020, Ireland recorded its first case of Covid.[4] Following the outbreak in Ireland, St Patrick's festivities were curtailed. In his traditional speech for Ireland's national saint, Taoiseach Leo Varadkar[5] did not announce national festivities but national mobilization against Covid instead. This national day was "like no others":

> We all need to take steps to reduce close human contact. That is how the virus is spread. Not just at public gatherings or public places but also in our own homes . . . places of leisure and work. Large public gatherings are cancelled. All pubs and bars are shut.
> We have also asked people to curtail or cancel social gatherings like parties, weddings and other celebrations. I know these choices won't be easy, but they are necessary (Irish Government News Service, 2020a).

As human beings are generally said to be sociable and in need of social contacts and interactions, what Leo Varadkar demanded could only have a negative impact on Irish people's well-being and mental health. "This is the calm before the storm—before the surge", he further said. Retrospectively, those words would frame the state of fear and anxiety that people felt at the time. Then and in the future, though Coronavirus had and would have "a deep impact on jobs and economic activity", the Irish government would be there to support the people. "I know this is causing huge stress and anxiety to you and your families . . . on top of fear of the virus" (Irish Government News Service, 2020a). Before closing his Saint Patrick's message and addressing special thoughts to the world, the Taoiseach asked people to "look after [their] mental health and well-being as well as [their] physical health":

---

[3] See Philip Hyland, Frédérique Vallières *et al.* "Covid-19 mental health survey by Maynooth University and Trinity College finds high rates of anxiety". Maynooth: Maynooth University, 2020; Tom Burke, Anna Berry *et al.* "Increased psychological distress during Covid-19 and quarantine in Ireland: a national survey". *Journal of Clinical Medicine* 2020; 28; (9) 11.

[4] For a chronology of Covid-related events in Ireland, see Antoine Masdupuy, "La République d'Irlande face à l'épidémie de Coronavirus", *in Droit, santé et Société*, 2020/1, pp. 58–62. Paul Cullen, Dean Ruxton, Colm Keena, Amanda Ferguson, "Coronavirus: Man treated in Dublin hospital as officials trace contacts", *Irish Times*, 29 February 2020.

[5] The *Taoiseach* is the Irish and official name of the Prime Minister in the Republic of Ireland.

> The vast majority of us who contract COVID-19 will experience a mild illness ... but some will be hospitalised and sadly some people will die. [...] Some people watching will have seen their jobs lost ... businesses closed ... or their working hours reduced. More will be worried that this might happen to them too ... especially as we do not know when the Emergency will end (Irish Government News Service, 2020a)

In a follow-up analysis of the speech, journalist Miriam Lord contrasted the green lit Government buildings with the emptiness of the streets, the "silent night of that unforgettable national day" (Lord, 2020). She then wrote, framing the atmosphere of the time:

> For these are frightening times. People are scared. Worried about protecting themselves and the health of their loved ones and worried sick about what might happen if they can't work and pay the bills (Lord, 2020).

The Irish lockdown was about to become one of the most "stringent" lockdowns ever experienced among EU countries (Cullen, 2021). Though the pandemic had reached Ireland's shores and led to the first lockdown, life was not completely at a standstill. Political life was still active as Ireland had just come out of a General Election in the first few months of 2020, and its results came just a month before the Covid pandemic. After long uncertain weeks between February and June 2020 in which no government was formed, the country managed to form a coalition government composed of Fine Gael, Fianna Fáil, and the Greens.[6] They agreed on a *Programme of government* which called for changes in Irish society (Department of the Taoiseach, 2020). Experiencing the pandemic had led parties to re-assess priorities, and thus well-being was very much placed to the fore along other environmental issues. Has uncertainty about the future led to a new thinking on well-being for the twenty-first century[7]? In other words, did the prospect of a worldwide pandemic (after much environmental concern expressed by the new generations) lead to some rethinking as to what matters in Irish society? Did the pandemic make well-being a more pressing issue in Ireland? As the notion of well-being itself is present in a series of documents following the new coalition's programme, one might be tempted to

---

[6]Leo Varadkar (Fine Gael) was the Taoiseach of the Republic of Ireland between 2017 and 2020. The election of February 2020 was a three-party race: Sinn Fein got 24.5% of the votes, Fianna Fail 22%, and Fine Gael with 21% of the votes. 130 days after the general election, a coalition between Fianna Fail, Fine Gael, and the Greens was formed as a way to keep nationalist party Sinn Féin out of power, which came first as voters were dissatisfied with a lack of housing and a poor healthcare system. It was the first time in Irish history that the two centre-right parties entered government together. Under the deal, Micheál Martin became the Taoiseach and Leo Varadkar the Tánaiste or deputy prime minister. It was decided that the roles would be reversed in December 2022.

[7]"The economic outlook is uncertain and depends on factors including the possibility of new waves of the virus, the emergence of new virus mutations, the stringency and duration of continued and/or new containment measures, the success of measures in controlling the spread of the virus, effective vaccines being rolled out and the behavioural response of consumers and firms when the economy reopens etc". Those elements could all impact on the well-being of people (inc. hospitalizations) and contribute to that uncertainty about the future that was prevalent at the time. See Abian Garcia-Rodrigueza, Adele Bergina, Luke Rehillb, and Éamonn Sweeney, "Exploring the Impact of Covid-19 and Recovery Paths for the Economy", ESRI, Working Paper 706, August 2021, p. 2.

give a positive answer, particularly as well-being and Covid-19 seem to be combined as a reaction towards a more caring and healthy society. Infographics and surveys released by the Irish Central Statistics Office (CSO) during the pandemic also show that well-being has remained on the agenda along other issues such as the economy. However, one may note that well-being itself is not clearly defined nor considered for itself but as a solution to better allocate resources. Is that a new issue in Irish politics? Has Ireland become a more caring society? And, as the Taoiseach's Saint Patrick message and the successive publications have aimed at protecting the most vulnerable, can we assess the impact of Covid-19 on specific groups such as young people in Irish society?

5.4   Well-Being in Ireland: The Official View

During the pandemic crisis, in the wake of the government's programme, three main documents were published on well-being in Ireland. They all attest to a need to study and define well-being in Irish society. Following commitments made within the coalition's programme, the *First Report on a Well-Being Framework for Ireland* was published in July 2021 by the Department of the Taoiseach. One year on from the start of the pandemic, the 59-page document called for a rethinking of Ireland's policy on well-being. Alongside the Government's *First Report*, the National Economic and Social Council (NESC), an organization in charge of developing strategic policies in Ireland, published the results of a consultation about well-being entitled *Ireland's Well-Being Framework: Consultation Report*. Finally, a paper entitled *Budget 2021—Well-being and the measurement of broader living standards in Ireland* was also released by the Irish Department of Finance in October 2020 to review and to assess international best practices in measuring well-being, and the recipe for an Irish well-being indicator.[8]

The three documents insist on the need to move "from GDP to well-being" (Department of Finance, 2020, 5) and the concept of well-being and especially the well-being of citizens appears to have become central to all policies in Ireland. In that sense, they echo the *Programme for Government—Our Shared Future* with its insistence to "move beyond uniquely economic measures" (Department of the Taoiseach, 2020, 6) since "the limits of existing approaches, in economic, social and environmental terms have generated momentum to develop alternative measures

---

[8]Interestingly, the authors specified that its contents did not represent the views of the Department of Finance nor the Government's: "Unless explicitly referenced by Government decision, any proposal contained in this document does not represent Government policy and should not be represented as such. The analysis and views set out in this paper do not necessarily reflect the views of the Minister for Finance". Furthermore, well-being and living standards are used to refer to the same concept which introduces a bias into the document from the outset as well as important limitations: "For the purposes of this paper, the terms well-being and living standards will be used interchangeably to refer to the same concept" (Department of Finance, 2020 3).

of societal progress" (NESC, 2021, 6). Indeed, *Budget 2021—Well-being and the measurement of broader living standards* explains, in the section entitled "moving from GDP to well-being" (Department of Finance, 2020, 5), that economic development and growth experienced in Ireland since the Celtic Tiger in the 1990s and early 2000s no longer meant individual and/or societal well-being, and that happiness did not always match the wealth of a country. Indicators such as GDP or GNP "are distorted by globalisation and increasingly disconnected from effective trends in living standards". Thus, the three publications insist on the need to change the way well-being is measured and thought in Ireland.

> If the growth of economic output does not directly or indirectly improve living standards and well-being, then an alternative measure is necessary to ensure the drive for economic growth does not eclipse progress towards higher living standards for all. (Department of Finance, 2020, 6)[9] (Authors' emphasis)

In that sense, the documents align themselves to the international consensus on the limitations of traditional macroeconomic indicators to reflect societal progress.[10] The OECD work is very much present, especially the series, *How's Life*, published every 2 years. A dashboard with a set of indicators similar to the OECD was chosen in Ireland with the possibility of creating a well-being framework at government's level using data from the CSO (Department of Finance, 2020). In a nutshell, a dashboard tailored to the Irish context with specific elements that matter to Irish people will be implemented (Department of Finance, 2020, 8 and 10).[11]

However, if the well-being framework for Ireland is presented as a way to improve the lives of people:

> The Well-being Framework is an important and ambitious cross-government initiative that seeks to develop a multi-dimensional approach to understanding the impact of public policy, driven by a desire to understand and do better by people. (6)

NESC's *Ireland's Well-Being Framework* does acknowledge the importance and influence of the pandemic as a sort of instigator which pushed for a shift in perspective:

---

[9] See also "Firstly, they are disconnected from living conditions and in particular distributional outcomes and inequalities. Secondly, they do not reflect the enormous value of the environment or give any indication of the sustainability of current output or income—current patterns of resource use and economic activity generally are putting huge pressure on the planet in a way that threatens the ability to meet future needs. Policy-making that ignores these weaknesses and focuses solely on GDP and equivalent aggregate economic measures could, "drive activities which may have a negative impact on well-being in the long-term"" (Department of Taoiseach, 2021).

[10] Read as well Didier Blanchet et Marc Fleurbaey, "De quoi le PIB est la mesure et comment le dépasser", *La vie des idées*, février 2021, https://laviedesidees.fr/De-quoi-le-PIB-est-la-mesure-et-comment-le-depasser.html [last accessed 4 January 2022].

[11] For this matter, a working group was established to work on this framework, in association with government's departments, the NESC, the CSO, and members of civil societies. They met four times between March and June 2021, but until now, no minutes have been published. Does it mean that the interest for such a consultation has eroded?

The 2020 Programme for Government announced the intention to create a set of well-being indicators for use in driving policy and evaluating outcomes. It highlighted the potential of the COVID-19 pandemic to increase poverty and inequality and the potential role of well-being measurement to ensure a fair and balanced recovery. (6)

The study of these official documents suggests that the new Irish government in early 2020 was committed to offering a different approach to well-being definition and measurement, and was keen to take on board such a concept into its future policies. The fact that the new coalition's *Programme for Government: Our Shared Future* was initially published on 29 October 2020 and updated on 7 April 2021 does suggest that the pandemic and its subsequent lockdown did strengthen such commitments towards a more caring and sustainable Ireland. However, such a view would need to be nuanced as this shift towards well-being also appears to be oriented towards designing better public policies while providing a better and more careful and rational allocation of public resources as the following paragraph states:

Over time, it is intended that the Well-being Framework will be utilised in a systematic way across government policymaking, for example, in reporting progress, setting policy priorities, and as a complementary tool for evaluating policies and programmes. It will therefore work in tandem with other Government initiatives that enhance using limited public resources efficiently to deliver effective public services (e.g., performance budgeting and spending review process) and focus attention on questions around differences in people's experiences (e.g., equality budgeting). (Department of Taoiseach, 2021, p. 2). (Authors' emphasis)

5.5 Representing Well-Being in Ireland: The CSO's Analysis

During the pandemic, the Central Statistics Office (CSO), the State's official statistical agency, set up a Covid-19 information hub on their website. The hub aimed at reporting "on the changing state of aspects of Ireland's economy and society since the Covid-19 outbreak".[12] It presented a number of entries on various population groups, on schools, on the impact of Covid-19 on people's well-being as well as some more specific focus on economic life and Irish households' budgets. Nearly a year after the lockdown began in Ireland, the *Social Impact of Covid-19 survey* on well-being reported some negative impacts on Irish people. 57.1% of its respondents reported that "their mental health/well-being" had been negatively affected by the pandemic. It appeared as well that more than 40% of respondents rated their overall life satisfaction as low, "the highest rating for low" recorded and that the period had also a negative impact on younger adult respondents as they were 20.5% aged 18–34 to report being regularly downhearted or depressed in the 4 week period prior to interview. There was an age difference regarding mental health as it appears that

---

[12] *Covid-19 Information Hub*. https://www.cso.ie/en/releasesandpublications/ep/p-Covid19/Covid-19informationhub/ [last accessed 15 April 2022].

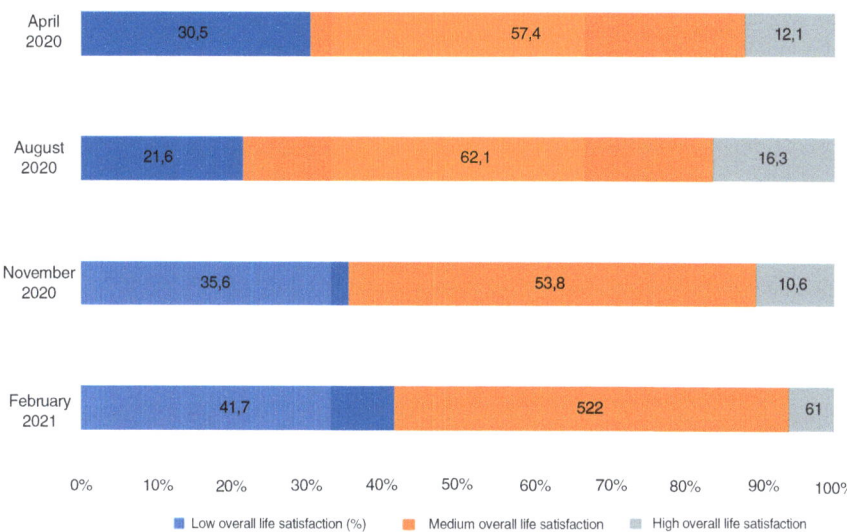

Fig. 5.1 Overall life satisfaction in Ireland (selected dates). Source: Central Statistics Office, Covid-19 Information Hub, 12 April 2022

only one-third (32.4%) of people aged 70 and over saw their mental health/well-being negatively affected by the pandemic in the February 2021 survey (CSO, 2021).

There was an increase between the various surveys in the number of people feeling downhearted or depressed most of the time, and a gender difference as more women, in proportion, reported feeling lonely all or most of the time than men (16.9–9.2%). It also appears that the level of satisfaction with life in general has declined since the first series, and the February 2021 survey records the "lowest overall life satisfaction scores" since 2013 (see Fig. 5.1).[13] The low satisfaction score follows the imposition and easing of restrictions on the Irish population. For example, in August 2020, it was only the very beginning of the second wave of the pandemic. Though Taoiseach Micheál Martin announced that face coverings were mandatory in shops (Irish Government News Service, 2020c),[14] Irish people remained quite optimistic during the summer 2020. With the return of restrictions, the low satisfaction rate rose to more than a third. On 19 October 2020, the Taoiseach announced that Ireland moved to level 5 of restrictions with schools and

---

[13] Late data from the CSO showed that 44.2% rated their overall life satisfaction as "high" in 2018 when Ireland's economic growth had recovered from the economic crisis. This latter period was marked by a lower rate at 31.1% in 2013. See infographics on CSO website at https://www.cso.ie/en/releasesandpublications/ep/p-Covid19/Covid-19informationhub/socialandwell-being/socialimpactofCovid-19survey/ [last accessed 15 April 2022].

[14] Face coverings were already compulsory for public transport.

childcare services remaining open. However, on 24 November 2020, speaking to the *Dáil*, Micheál Martin stated the difficulty of families of dealing with remote teaching and remote work:

> Almost one fifth of women with children in school were unable to work with school closures, and a much larger number of parents faced increased pressure and limits on their ability to work (Irish Government News Service, 2020e).

To that must be added a higher loneliness score for most people, especially during the pandemic and the imposition of restrictions on the Irish population. Furthermore, 10 months after the beginning of the crisis, there was also an increase in the number of people feeling downhearted or depressed. The CSO thus states that "in November 2020, 11.5% of respondents reported that they felt downhearted or depressed *All or Most of the time*, double the equivalent rate in April 2020 (5.5%). In February 2021, this rate increased to 15.1% (almost three times the April 2020 rate)". Moreover, the feeling of being lonely also increased from the first survey, though it remained rather unchanged between November 2020 and February 2021. In that same survey, there is a gender difference as women report lower well-being indicators than men. Younger respondents also reported lower well-being scores, while there also appears to be a high compliance with government's advice and guidelines (CSO, 2021). Then, there is also a feeling of despair about the current restrictions and some pessimism as to the future, and a widespread feeling that life will not go back to normal till much later. Such results are likely to be similar with other studies in other European countries regarding loneliness or uncertainty about the future (including what will happen with restrictions in the coming months).

5.6   Impact of the Crisis on Well-Being: The Case of Young People

The *First Report on a Well-Being Framework for Ireland* stresses the consequences on people and sectors with a particular focus on sectors and group of population:

> Those working in labour-intensive customer-facing sectors, who tend to be lower paid, younger, less skilled and cannot as easily work remotely, had their jobs impacted most heavily, and require the greatest support in moving to new areas of opportunity. (Department of Taoiseach, 2021, p. 7)

Since the global spread of Covid-19, there has been substantial research conducted to identify the immediate and possible long-term impacts on young people.[15]

---

[15] Similar findings on other groups among the population have been found. According to recent studies, the Covid-19 pandemic has tended to worsen the disadvantages experienced by migrants and ethnic minorities in Ireland. See McGinnity et al., (2020). Covid-19 and non-Irish nationals in Ireland [Report]. ESRI and Department of Children, Equality, Disability, Integration and Youth. https://doi.org/10.26504/bkmnext404 [last accessed 24 April 2022]; Hennessy, (2021, January 6). The Impacts of Covid-19 on Ethnic Minority and Migrant Groups in Ireland. National Economic &

International research shows that, though young people were initially supposed to be the least affected by the Covid-19 infection as few of them developed severe forms, it appears that they were inversely the most affected by its consequences, notably in the areas of mental health and education. The situation in Ireland is similar. Several reports and online surveys demonstrated that the Covid-19 pandemic had negative effects on young people's health and well-being, especially amongst marginalized groups (Irish Government News Service, 2020d) and young people who were already deemed "most at risk" as they "became the most disconnected from youth services and supports as a result of Covid-19" (Youth Council of Ireland, 2020).

Indeed, on 12 March 2020, Saint Patrick's festivities were not only curtailed but Taoiseach Leo Varadkar also announced the closing of all schools, colleges, and childcare facilities. With "the mandatory order for people to stay at home announced on 28 March 2020, educational facilities remained closed until August 2020". Moreover, despite the different measures implemented during fall 2020, schools, which were open between August and December 2020, did not reopen after Christmas 2021 and remained closed until 1 March 2021 for junior infants to second class and Leaving Certificate students (about 320,000 pupils). For higher education, the situation was even worse, from March 2020, most lectures and classes were online (as they were in other higher education institutions across Europe). This was also the case for the majority of higher education institutions for the academic year of 2020–21. The situation only got back to normal for the academic year of 2021–22, that is to say, after one and a half years of remote teaching.[16]

A report released by the Economic and Social Research Institute (ESRI), an Irish organization in charge of analysing the Irish economy and promoting social progress, looked at the impact of Covid-19 on children and young people. Launching the report, Minister for Children and Youth Affairs once again acknowledged the impact of Covid-19 on children and young people, stating that it had not been even across all sectors, and that its impacts could be of two sorts: economic (unemployment, and some effects on housing through rent) and social (to be cut off from friends, mental health impacts, and other elements brought by cumulative disadvantages).[17] It was thus shown, according to the Minister, that Covid-19 had an impact on family relationships, on social life, on existing inequalities which had been exacerbated by closures of schools and universities, and on health and well-being.

Social Council, Research Series, Paper No.18. http://files.nesc.ie/nesc_research_series/research_series_paper_18_Covid19Migrants.pdf [last accessed 24 April 2022].

[16] During that period, especially during the second lockdown, some buildings in colleges and universities remained open such as libraries.

[17] This report was presented during one of the webinars the Economic and Social Research Institute organized during the lockdown. Webinar: Implications of the Covid-19 pandemic for policy in relation to children and young people—20 July 2020. Merike Darmody, Emer Smyth and Helen Russell, *The Implications of the Covid-19 Pandemic for Policy in Relation to Children and Young People: a Research Review*, ESRI, Research Review, number 94, July 2020. DOI: https://doi.org/10.26504/sustat94

The Minister also referred to a study, entitled *How is your head, Young voices during Covid-19* written by his department (for children, disability, equality, and integration) and SpunOut.[18] The report shows how young people struggled with being separated from their friends and faced significant mental health impacts as a result of Covid-19 and its restrictions. During its online presentation, its two researchers (Emer Smyth and Helen Russell) presented their work insisting on the online dimension of the survey with some of its limitations (not everyone is included, not representative of the whole population) while acknowledging that they also work with the CSO *Social Impact Covid* survey. The various consequences of Covid-19 were its implications on health (disruption of care in hospitals and impact on physical education in schools, for example) with an impact on all groups, but weighing more strongly on disadvantaged people. Though Covid-19 and the restrictions also gave way to positive outcomes (more time spent with family) with some difficulties linked to overcrowding (as it caused necessary living arrangements, including parenting challenges, while in some instances, it also led unfortunately to even domestic violence), it also imposed a double burden on parents (in Ireland and internationally) as they had to combine working from home and homeschooling, with a more severe impact on women than men.

They also referred to international research which has shown the impact of Covid-19 on well-being and mental health, showing a rise in anxiety levels and depression due to some social isolation. Indeed, the online consultation also demonstrated that almost every young people experienced difficulties, both major and minor (Department for Children, Disability, Equality and Integration and SpunOut, 2020, 13). More worrying, almost 10% of the respondents could not name any positive points during this period (6). The answer to the question "What have you been finding hard during Covid-19?" clearly shows the negative effects on young people's health and well-being. The respondents indicated "overthinking, concern, worry, anxiety, depression and a sense of utter hopelessness" (6). Over a third of young people (35%[19]) stated that "missing friends was the hardest thing with which they had been forced to cope with" (14), friendship being of utmost importance at this age. The online consultation also clearly showed a feeling of cabin fever or confinement present in many answers (350 respondents) (15):[20]

---

[18] An online consultation of young people between 15 and 24 took place during the summer 2020. The goal was to better understand how young people experienced Covid-19 in Ireland. 2173 valid responses were used for this survey (Department for children, disability, equality and integration and SpunOut 2020).

[19] more women (38%) than men (31%), travelers: 40%.

[20] This ranged from those who were only somewhat fed up about having restrictions placed on their movements to those who found themselves completely trapped in highly dysfunctional domestic situations. Young women and Travellers were more likely to report cabin fever. Many of the over-18 s who had been forced to return to live in the family home, commented on losing their independence and adult freedoms, which sometimes led to a strain on family relations (Department for Children, Disability, Equality and Integration and SpunOut, 2020, 15).

> I feel totally purposeless, demotivated and lost during this time, I feel like most of the activities I do during the day are simply day fillers rather than anything I actually enjoy, I can't drive so I truly am stuck in my house which is in a rural area with a scarcity of services/facilities. All of this has contributed to major hardship on my mental health—Female, 21, rural location. (Irish Government News Service, 2020d)

This report confirms what both Taoisigh said during the pandemic. For example, on 1 May 2020, in a heart touching speech, the Taoiseach reasserted the depressed atmosphere in Ireland and spoke about Jessica: "A letter from Jessica, who is a wheelchair user, who feels an enormous cloud of loneliness around her" or about Phil: "A letter from Phil, a pensioner living alone, who admits to struggling with the isolation and lack of human contact and whose mental health is starting to suffer" (Irish Government News Service, 2020b). Clearly, the nation feels depressed as this was clearly stated by the CSO surveys about mental health and Covid-19.

To alleviate this problem, on 8 June 2020, Taoiseach Varadkar and Minister Daly launched an online service, CAMHS Connect, to provide online support and telepsychiatry for remote patients and young patients. The Taoiseach explained:

> COVID-19 has brought home something we have always known, that maintaining and improving our mental health is an essential part of our well-being. Positive mental health enhances our ability to cope with the stresses of everyday life, and makes us more engaged, productive and happy citizens. Now more than ever, we realise the importance of looking after our mental health. Back in 2012 the funding for Mental Health in our country was €711m. Today it is just over a billion euro, because the Government recognises how much it matters to our health and well-being. Over the past few years we have been developing new online responses to complement existing mental health care in Ireland, long before we had ever heard of COVID-19 (Irish Government News Service 2020b).

Once again, mental health and well-being are associated, being an "essential part", if not synonymous.

According to second researcher, Helen Russell, Covid had an impact on formal learning with educational disruption, but also underlined a lack of research on students, and also some negative effects on special education students (SEN) and migrant children. Indeed, almost one in five (18%) worried about their education, particularly those aged 18 or over (28% vs 18% for under 18).[21] The respondents mentioned missing going to school/college. They were worried for their education and also needed "having daily connections with peers and teachers" (Department for Children, Disability, Equality and Integration and SpunOut, 2020). Obviously, "online learning was deemed a poor substitute, especially for those with hardware and internet access issues" (14). Many young people have also lost out in missing "rites of passage" of school such as sitting key examinations, finishing the school year, graduating from school or college, participating in youth exchanges or overseas trips (16).

Finally, youth unemployment was a true problem, particularly as youth-friendly sectors (retail, hospitality) were among the hardest hit sectors, and young people

---

[21] Again more women 23% than men 13%.

were over-represented in terms of job losses. Indeed, unemployment skyrocketed during the pandemic especially for young people:

> The second distinctive impact is the disproportionate one on younger workers. When PUP [Pandemic Unemployment Payment] recipients are included, the unemployment rate in the 15-to-24 age cohort rose to 46 per cent in the fourth quarter of last year, compared with a total unemployment rate of 19.8 per cent. In part, this is because of the higher incidence of youth employment in the contact-intensive sectors of the economy—often in part-time or entry-level jobs.[22]

This rise of youth unemployment had two consequences. First, many respondents expressed worries about their financial situation: Would they be able to afford college the following year? Would there be employment options in their chosen field if there was an economic downturn? Also, some expressed frustration about not being eligible for the Covid-19 Pandemic Unemployment Payment (Department for Children, Disability, Equality and Integration and SpunOut, 2020, 17). For example:

> I was forced to drop out of college … I relied on a grant and normally had to work another job over summer to pay rent in Dublin. I had to quit my jobs because there weren't enough hours and I can't get jobseekers assistance as I'm under 24 and I'm not eligible. (The state assumes you're financially dependent on family if you're under 24, but that's not reality for many of us.) Female, 20, urban location. (Irish Government News Service, 2020d)

Some students stopped working and became isolated or, worse, experienced poverty during the pandemic (Youth Council of Ireland (NYCI), 2020, 2). To remedy such concerns, on 19 October 2020, the Taoiseach announced financial subsidies such as PUP and EWSS [Employment Wage Subsidy Scheme] would be improved. Secondly, in such a context, long-term effects (such as higher rates of drop-outs or impacts on learning) are not fully known, and show that often in periods of recession, it is all the more difficult for those entering employment to start in life.[23] Moreover, young people making their transition to the labour market were hit even harder, particularly as emigration was no longer possible because of the restrictions on travelling and moving countries during the peak of the pandemic.[24]

Following the government's commitment, the CSO has released a series of indicators which presented the state of well-being in Ireland in its *Social Impact of*

---

[22] Paschal Donohoe TD (2021, March 4). "The Pandemic: One Year On". Speech by Minister for Finance Mr. Paschal Donohoe TD, Economic and Social Research Institute, https://www.gov.ie/en/speech/ad527-the-pandemic-one-year-on-speech-by-the-minister-for-finance-mr-paschal-donohoe-td-economic-and-social-research-institute-march-4th-2021/ [last accessed 4 March 2022].

[23] This inability to gain experience means that young people find it harder to get a first-time experience on the job market. They could face some extra difficulties to move on to better paid jobs once they have acquired some work experience. In that sense, it would represent a form of disadvantage compared to other groups.

[24] The report refers to the release valve of migration (outward migration), no longer possible during Covid and lockdown (as a difference with the Global financial crisis—"for pressure in the Irish labour market with large levels of emigration synonymous with recessions in the country")— Matthew Allen-Coghlan and Petros Varthalitis, Comparing two recessions in Ireland: Global Financial Crisis vs Covid-19, ESRI Research Notes 2020/4/1, https://doi.org/10.26504/rn20200401, p. 8.

Covid-19 survey series (see Infographics and link to CSO website). Across a wide range of indicators, Covid-19 has had an impact on people's well-being, with some people more affected than others, as in any country despite numerous initiatives implemented by the Irish government and the civil society. Apart from health issues, the aforementioned studies have shown that young people had been deeply affected by Covid-19. The pandemic shows a series of cumulative disadvantages which has also shown that existing inequalities were reinforced during Covid, especially on the labour market, as sectors traditionally hiring many young people such as hospitality and retail closed during lockdowns, leading to some negative social and economic consequences.

5.7 Conclusion

At the time of writing [May 2022], it remains quite difficult to assess the full well-being costs of Covid-19 in Ireland and on Irish people. The effects of the Covid-19 pandemic on each country and its citizens will be long-felt and will remain as one milestone in the history of each individual. Irish authorities have fought the unequal consequences of the pandemic on people and sectors, while simultaneously trying to improve well-being. Whether or not they have succeeded in their endeavour remains hard to assess without the full benefit of hindsight. Inequalities existed prior to Covid-19, and for young people, the pandemic has served to expose a whole range of inequalities and has also exacerbated vulnerabilities whether in terms of mental health or in education (young people were worried about the uncertainty of their exams, the conditions of the reopening of institutions, no access to the support schools provide, *etc.*). Covid-19 has also had adverse effects on the employment situation of young adults (temporary lay-off or loss of employment) and has delayed entry on the Irish labour market.

However, the pandemic does reveal that Irish authorities may have realized that Ireland, facing multiple challenges, was at a crossroads. Irish authorities at last asserted that, with the importance of multinationals in the country, well-being could no longer be measured on GDP terms only—this measure being distorted—but needed to rest on a wide range of indicators to fully grasp the impacts of progress on Irish society. However virtuous those statements are in the different reports previously studied, it is important to note that the issue of value for money dominates as successive Irish governments work on a well-being dashboard. To create Ireland's own dashboard, Irish authorities considered different well-being frameworks among OECD countries with a particular focus on New Zealand. The implementation of the well-being framework should follow suit in the coming months and years. As Ireland and the world emerge from the pandemic, it remains to be seen to what extent such commitments to well-being will top the Irish government's agenda and how it will be embedded in future policies. In its September 2021 report on the Well-being Framework, the Oireachtas, the national Parliament of Ireland, called for its cooptation into the consultative process, an institutional structure dedicated to well-being, and an increased parliamentary scrutiny over policy choices and the allocation of public resources.[25] Successive governmental and institutional publications mentioned previously show a definite commitment to well-being in Ireland. However, communication towards the general public seems to be lacking. A survey of Irish newspaper articles does not reveal a huge number of articles on the latest well-being initiatives. Well-being in Ireland would therefore greatly gain from a widespread communication in the media. Such awareness on well-being would encourage all people and communities to engage further through debates and discussions on important issues such as education, sustainability, and work which matter for younger generations.

References

Banks, J., Fancourt, D., & Xiaowei, X. (2021). Mental health and the COVID-19 pandemic. In J. F. Helliwell, R. Layard, J. Sachs, & J.-E. De Neve (Eds.), *World happiness report 2021* (pp. 107–130). Sustainable development solutions network.

Central Statistics Office. (2021, February). *Press statement - Social impact of Covid-19 survey February 2021: Well-being*. CSO. https://www.cso.ie/en/csolatestnews/pressreleases/2021 pressreleases/pressstatementsocialimpactofCovid-19surveyfebruary2021well-being/

Cullen, P. (2021, May 7). Ireland had EU's most stringent lockdown this year, analysis finds. *The Irish Times* https://www.irishtimes.com/news/health/ireland-had-eu-s-most-stringent-lock down-this-year-analysis-finds-1.4557746

Department for Children, Disability, Equality and Integration, & SpunOut. (2020, October). How is your head, Young voices during Covid-19. *Report of a national consultation with young people on mental health and well-being*. https://assets.gov.ie/91225/d2c21ebd-09de-4424-b9fb-ddf0 b404724f.pdf

Department of Finance. (2020, October). *Well-being and the measurement of broader living standards in Ireland*. https://www.gov.ie/en/publication/70874-well-being-and-the-measure ment-of-broader-living-standards-in-ireland/

Department of Taoiseach. (2020, October 29). *Programme for Government: Our shared future*. https://www.gov.ie/en/publication/7e05d-programme-for-government-our-shared-future/.

Department of Taoiseach. (2021, July). *First report on well-being framework for Ireland July 2021*. https://www.gov.ie/en/press-release/fb19a-first-report-on-well-being-framework-for-ireland-july-2021/

Economic & Social Research Institute. (2021, June 21). *Budget perspectives 2022 webinar: Covid-19 and the Irish welfare system*. https://www.youtube.com/watch?v=XHtPMm9J-GM

Hennessy, Ó. (2021, January 6). *The impacts of Covid-19 on ethnic minority and migrant groups in Ireland*. National economic and social council, research series, Paper No.18. http://files.nesc.ie/ nesc_research_series/research_series_paper_18_Covid19Migrants.pdf

Houses of the Oireachtas, Parliamentary Budget Office. (2021, September 15). *A well-being framework for Ireland - The parliamentary perspective*, Pub. 22. https://data.oireachtas.ie/ie/

---

[25] Houses of the Oireachtas, Parliamentary Budget Office (2021, September 15). *A Well-being Framework for Ireland—the Parliamentary Perspective*, Pub. 22. Retrieved May 8, 2022, from https://data.oireachtas.ie/ie/oireachtas/parliamentaryBudgetOffice/2021/2021-09-15_a-well-being-framework-for-ireland-the-parliamentary-perspective_en.pdf

oireachtas/parliamentaryBudgetOffice/2021/2021-09-15_a-well-being-framework-for-ireland-the-parliamentary-perspective_en.pdf

Irish Government News Service. (2020a, March 17). *National address by the Taoiseach, St Patrick's Day.* https://www.gov.ie/en/speech/72f0d9-national-address-by-the-taoiseach-st-patricks-day/

Irish Government News Service. (2020b, May 1). *Statement of An Taoiseach, Leo Varadkar T.D., Update on Covid-19 emergency.* https://merrionstreet.ie/en/News-Room/News/Statement_of_An_Taoiseach_Leo_Varadkar_T_D_Update_on_COVID-19_Emergency_.html

Irish Government News Service. (2020c, August 4). *Speech by An Taoiseach, Micheál Martin TD, Post Cabinet Briefing, 4* August 2020. https://merrionstreet.ie/en/News-Room/Speeches/Speech_by_An_Taoiseach_Micheal_Martin_TD_Post_Cabinet_Briefing_4_August_2020.html

Irish Government News Service. (2020d, October 5). *Minister O'Gorman launches the publication of 'How's Your Head – Young Voices during Covid-19', a national consultation with young people on mental health and well-being during Covid-19.* https://merrionstreet.ie/en/Category-Index/Health/minister_o'gorman_launches_the_publication_of_'how's_your_head_–_young_voices_during_Covid-19'_a_national_consultation_with_young_people_on_mental_health_and_well-being_during_Covid-19.161497.shortcut.html

Irish Government News Service. (2020e, November 24). *Dáil Speech by An Taoiseach Micheál Martin on Covid-19.* https://merrionstreet.ie/en/News-Room/Speeches/Dail_Speech_by_An_Taoiseach_Micheal_Martin_on_Covid-19.html

Kelly, B. D. (2020). Impact of Covid-19 on mental health in Ireland: Evidence to date. *Irish Medical Journal, 113*(10), 1–6.

Lord, M. (2020, March 18). Desperate times require extraordinary lines as Leo finds right words. *The Irish Times.* https://www.irishtimes.com/news/politics/miriam-lord-desperate-times-require-extraordinary-lines-as-leo-finds-right-words-1.4205660

McGinnity, F., Russell, H., Privalko, I., & Enright, S. (2020). *COVID-19 and non-Irish nationals in Ireland [Report].* ESRI and Department of Children, Equality, Disability, Integration and Youth. https://doi.org/10.26504/bkmnext404.

NESC. (2021, July). *Ireland's well-being framework: Consultation report* (N° 155). http://files.nesc.ie/nesc_reports/en/155_WBF.pdf

Okabe-Miyamoto, K., & Lyubomirsky, S. (2021). Social connection and well-being during COVID-19. In J. F. Helliwell, R. Layard, J. Sachs, & J.-E. De Neve (Eds.), *World happiness report 2021* (pp. 131–152). Sustainable development solutions network.

Schmidtke, J., Hetschko, C., Schöb, R., Stephan, G., Eid, M., & Lawes, M. (2021). *The effects of the Covid-19 pandemic on the mental health and subjective well-being of workers: An event study based on High-Frequency Panel Data.* IZA Discussion Papers (N° 14638; IZA Discussion Papers). Institute of Labor Economics (IZA). https://ideas.repec.org/p/iza/izadps/dp14638.html

World Health Organization. (2020, March 11). *WHO Director-General's opening remarks at the media briefing on COVID-19—11* March 2020. https://www.who.int/director-general/speeches/detail/who-director-general-s-opening-remarks-at-the-media-briefing-on-Covid-19%2D%2D-11-march-2020

Youth Council of Ireland (NYCI). (2020). NYCI research shows Covid-19 pandemic impacting most severely on 'at risk' youth. *National Youth Council of Ireland.* https://www.youth.ie/articles/Covidreport/

Vanessa Boullet is an associate professor at the University of Lorraine. Her research focuses on Irish studies, and on the interactions between economy, society, and politics. Her thesis entitled "Planning in Ireland (1958–1972), methodologies and mythology of economic modernisation" was awarded the Prix Richelieu by the Chancellerie des Universités de Paris in 2009. She has developed an interest in the impact of multinationals on the Irish economy and its uneven development. She also tries to develop research in Business and Foreign Languages departments in France and she is a member of the editorial board of the journal *Revue International des Langues Appliquées Etrangères*.

Julien Guillaumond is a lecturer in English at Clermont-Auvergne University. He holds a Ph.D. in Irish studies from Sorbonne University on social and economic inequalities in the twentieth century Ireland. He is a member of the research lab Communication and Sociétés, and is currently part of the GIS EIRE research network. His research interests include citizenship and inequality issues in contemporary societies as well as various aspects of Irish political, economic, and social history. He is currently working on diaspora issues in Ireland and France, together with identity representations and development with a particular focus on Irish tourism and nation branding.

Part II
The Impact of Covid-19 on Education

Chapter 6
Challenges to Higher Education at the Start of the Pandemic with a Comparative Focus on the UK and Hong Kong

Iside Costantini

Abstract This chapter examines the Covid impact on university students in the UK and Hong Kong and assesses the inequalities at stake concerning well-being whilst emphasizing the unequal costs within the higher education and research sector among students, faculties, and institutions. Hong Kong as a previous British colony has built its higher education system on the British model and although it carries some distinctive local features, the two may be comparable in terms of structure, delivery, and expectations.

To begin with, it will draw on a definition of the predominant framework of Anglo-Saxon well-being and examine how this applies to education and crisis management. Secondly, it will evaluate through reports from major institutions (ONS, OECD, European University Association and Universities UK (Universities UK represents 140 universities in England, Scotland, Wales, and Northern Ireland and works with the government, universities, and stakeholders to continue improving the UK's education sector)), which were conducted from 2020 to 2021, the global impact of the pandemic on higher education learning (the virtual experience) as well as the perception of programmes of education by staff and students.

Thirdly, this chapter will attempt to reflect on inequalities caused by these new forms of learning patterns which could also help bring in more equality (for instance, time flexibility, less transport, lower spending on accommodation for students).

In the short term, this renewed approach to teaching may appear to be positive with the development of hybrid forms of teaching, more online courses, and an overall cheaper operational model. In the long run, if this situation became more recurrent, this could lead to new challenges and create inequalities between graduates if not a gap which would be difficult to bridge for the concerned age groups and have an impact on the educational systems of both the UK and Hong Kong.

I. Costantini (✉)
Université Sorbonne Nouvelle, Paris, France
e-mail: iside.costantini@sorbonne-nouvelle.fr

© The Author(s), under exclusive license to Springer Nature Switzerland AG 2022   95
L. Dalingwater et al. (eds.), *The Unequal Costs of Covid-19 on Well-being in Europe*,
Human Well-Being Research and Policy Making,
https://doi.org/10.1007/978-3-031-14425-7_6

6.1   Introduction

This chapter examines the Covid impact on university students in the UK and Hong Kong and assesses the inequalities at stake concerning well-being whilst emphasizing the unequal costs within the higher education and research sector among students, faculties, and institutions. Hong Kong as a previous British colony has built its higher education system on the British model and although it carries some distinctive local features, the two may be comparable in terms of structure, delivery, and expectations.

To begin with, it will draw on a definition of the predominant framework of Anglo-Saxon well-being and examine how this applies to education and crisis management. Secondly, it will evaluate through reports from major institutions (ONS, OECD, European University Association, and Universities UK[1]), which were conducted from 2020 to 2021, the global impact of the pandemic on higher education learning (the virtual experience) as well as the perception of programmes of education by staff and students.

Thirdly, this chapter will attempt to reflect on inequalities caused by these new forms of learning patterns which could also help bring in more equality (for instance, time flexibility, less transport, lower spending on accommodation for students).

In the short term, this renewed approach to teaching may appear to be positive with the development of hybrid forms of teaching, more online courses, and an overall cheaper operational model. In the long run, if this situation became more recurrent, this could lead to new challenges and create inequalities between graduates if not a gap which would be difficult to bridge for the concerned age groups and have an impact on the educational systems of both the UK and Hong Kong.

6.2   Definition of Anglo-Saxon Well-being

Research on well-being was first undertaken in the Anglo-Saxon world and referred to under the term "subjective well-being" (SWB). The birth of the scientific review *Journal of Happiness Studies (An Interdisciplinary Forum on Subjective Well-being)* in 2000 reveals to what extent a new field of study has developed. Over half of the research registered in the World Database of Happiness (based in the Erasmus Happiness Economics Research Organization of Erasmus University Rotterdam) directed by well-being specialist Ruut Veenhoven has been undertaken in the US. However, this database which helped institutionalize a new field of research tends to include mostly English language publications as over half of the surveys were conducted in the US (Pawin, 2014, p. 274). Methodology was initially based on

---

[1] Universities UK represents 140 universities in England, Scotland, Wales, and Northern Ireland and works with the government, universities, and stakeholders to continue improving the UK's education sector.

"hedonic level of affect" that is "the degree to which affective experience is dominated by pleasantness during a certain period" (Veenhoven & Brulé, 2014, p. 38). According to those studies, well-being is considered as part of the emotional aspect of a subject, as one experiences it, beyond any other analytical or cognitive process. The other types of studies were based on contentment or satisfaction: "the degree to which an individual perceives his conscious aims to be achieved" (Veenhoven & Brulé, 2014, p. 38). Well-being is here understood as self-perception of one's achievements. The overall result would sum up the degree of adequation between the representations of reality and experience (Pawin, 2014, pp. 275–76).

According to the *Stanford Encyclopedia of Philosophy*, well-being "is most commonly used in philosophy to describe what is non-instrumentally or ultimately good for a person". The question of what well-being consists in is of importance in moral philosophy, especially in the case of utilitarianism, according to which well-being is to be maximized (Coron & Dalingwater, 2017, p. 11). It has taken on some economic characteristics linked to the importance of prosperity notably in the US, for instance, where the idea of well-being has a special resonance with the Declaration of Independence which states that the pursuit of happiness is one of Americans' inalienable rights (Coron & Dalingwater, 2017, p. 15). It seems that in the build up of American consumerism, the idea of purchasing goods to make oneself happy was largely predominant (Gorge et al., 2015, p. 112). Bryan Smith further accounts for a new correlation between well-being, purchasing power, and ownership.

> While American policymakers have consistently used happiness rhetoric and a specific notion of virtue to promote an ownership model of well-being, this may well have the opposite effect and make citizens feel unhappy if they fail to achieve accession to ownership (Coron & Dalingwater, 2017, p. 9)

In the UK, well-being has more recently been adjusted by policymakers to the neoliberal model of capitalism (Coron & Dalingwater, 2017, pp. 15–16). According to Dalingwater's cross-examination of well-being, the Whitehall Well-being Working Group (2006) statement of common understanding established among all government departments in the UK is based on "subjective well-being" that includes satisfying basic needs, fulfilling personal goals, developing a sense of purpose, having a participatory role in society, enjoying supportive personal relationships, being involved in empowered communities, and benefiting from an attractive environment (Coron & Dalingwater, 2017, pp. 112–113).

There is a consensus that well-being is relevant to students in higher education. University students are not just seeking financially secure employment opportunities and careers; in many countries, they rate well-being as more important than money because they desire to lead meaningful lives and not only have a successful career (Tay, 2021, p. 461). The Hong Kong Quality of Life which has been measured by the Chinese University of Hong Kong since 2003 revealed that Hong Kong people considered good health, peace of mind, and money as key to happiness and desired a better living environment, placing education as a key to success (Chan et al., 2005). The Covid-19 pandemic has exacerbated pre-existing trends leading to lower well-being in a context of economic uncertainty, social division and unrest, isolation, technological pressure, and unequal access to education in a changing environment.

6.3   Education and Crisis Management

Many articles have been written on how to maintain levels of well-being during a crisis and conclude that it is the responsibility of various actors (Brazeau et al., 2020, p. 688). "The Covid-19 pandemic has shaken the key assumptions and beliefs that serve as the foundation of higher education" (Brazeau et al., 2020, p. 688). It has continued to blur barriers between work and home activities (WHO, 2022), enabling one to establish priorities between both whilst gaining in efficiency.

Besides innovation and creativity, strong leading teams among faculty members and the flexibility of students appear as essential components to help navigate through the current health crisis (Brazeau et al., 2020, p. 689). These capacities may have contributed to strengthening the whole work community (improved work practices, spreading innovative methods, enhanced efficiency and cohesiveness). Indeed, according to an ONS report *Coronavirus and the impact on measures of UK government education output: March 2020 to February 2021*, "repeated changes to schooling policies during the coronavirus pandemic and the need to measure education output as consistently as possible have required us to keep innovating to ensure measurement keeps up with developments in schools" (Wales, 2021). This shows the positive and regenerative outcome that may derive from a crisis in terms of reinventing approaches and methods.

Crises are "acute, public, arduous threats to an organization and its stakeholders" (König et al., 2020, p. 130). In the case of the Covid pandemic, governments worldwide were concerned by maintaining stability and reorganizing social and economic activities through the rapid implementation of new rules. For the academic staff, there was little preparation to switch to a new system of teaching which consisted in maintaining usual activities and interaction online. To achieve this change within a short lapse of time, capacities and stamina to invest oneself into a new form of teaching were crucial to keep the institutions operational and the extent to which some were successful may have impacted personal well-being of staff and opened up new possibilities as a whole, while discouraging others in their search for a new equilibrium in their work-life balance. It has been well documented[2] how working from home may have blurred barriers and increased workload and stress levels thus leading to more burnouts among staff and students in schools and faculties. "Resilience, or the capacity to cope with stressors, can be linked to job

[2] A report from the World Health Organization (2022) says working from home can blur the boundaries and incurs longer working hours than before for individuals. Besides some people telework from difficult conditions, working from the same place where they relax. The blurred boundaries of home mean that sick teleworkers simply continue working and are expected to join meetings as usual, a phenomena known as "sickness presenteeism".

satisfaction, burnout and well-being" and these three aspects of resilience which are linked to the context can be seen as "processes with which the individual interacts within a broader social ecology" (Ainsworth & Oldfield, 2019, p. 2).

According to McNamara, communication between leaders in times of crisis is essential to reflect the concerted and combined efforts within an enterprise, embracing similar culture and values (7). An organization will only be able to move forward and maintain its unity after a crisis if it is able to re-connect and approach in a balanced way a new post-crisis environment (McNamara, 2021, p. 8). McNamara similarly concludes that by moving away from the immediate situation, "communities in Higher Education may be able to respond and progress in the face of tensions by engaging in a frank and open reflective discourse to recognise and expose shared frailties within structural processes and systems of operation and practice, in the knowledge that naming frailty is not equal to weakness, but rather acts to stimulate communal resilience" (McNamara, 2021, p. 10). Academia can learn from examining the recent process of change it has undergone and strengthen its collegiality by working on commonly acknowledged delivery failures and better prepare for the future despite unforeseen developments. According to a report *Covid's Lessons for Global Higher Education*, there could be a risk if institutions "overfocus on the short-term effects of the pandemic and satisfy themselves with a return to 'normal' instead of reshaping higher education for long-term resilience", by putting in place new practices acquired during the pandemic (Salmi, 2020, p. 13).

6.4   Covid Impact on University Students Through Surveys

Reports from the ONS, Universities UK, and European University Association examine and assess through surveys the impact of the pandemic on higher education learning and perception of programmes by students and staff. A study collecting data from 2707 university students in France, Germany, Russia, and the UK (Plakhotnik et al., 2021) examined how student perceptions of their degree completion and future job prospects during the pandemic impacted their well-being and concluded on the importance of mediation and university support provided by instructors and administration. Student well-being was affected by their short-term concerns for their degree completion but not by long-term job prospects. According to Plakhotnik et al., student well-being has been linked to "their engagement and performance in curricular [. . .] and extracurricular activities, intrinsic motivation, satisfaction, meaning making, and mental health".

The impact of the Covid pandemic on course content and learning patterns was overall perceived as negative by students in the UK and Hong Kong because the shift to an online version no longer met the expectations of the original format in terms of presentation and ease of assimilation. This feeling of dissatisfaction increased within six months and between the two ONS surveys held between the end of 2020 and early 2021 (Hamilton, 2021).

> A greater proportion of students reported being dissatisfied or very dissatisfied with their academic experience since the start of the autumn term (37%), than the 29% reporting the same at the end of November 2020 (20 to 25 November 2020). Of those who were dissatisfied with their academic experience, the most common reasons were learning delivery (75%) and quality of learning (71%). (ONS, 2020)

The traditional education mode, where the teacher continues teaching in a regular class setting that is broadcast live and can be retrieved later on, seems to be the most appreciated by students because this is closest to the format to which they are accustomed (UNESCO, 2020, p. 20). Undergraduates were not keen to partake in new methodology approaches where they would have to leave their comfort zone and interact more online.

A well-being survey held in Hong Kong shows that life satisfaction of the population decreased significantly between 2018 and 2020 over the years before and after social unrest, plus the outbreak of the coronavirus disease 2019 in Hong Kong (Wong et al., 2021). According to this source, the changes were more influenced by social unrest and Covid-19 related stressors than by personal ones.

In Hong Kong, the online teaching system was already in place by the end of 2019 because of earlier protests[3] (Jung et al., 2021, p. 6) and more generally, Asian students are known to be technical savvy so the online medium of instruction may have been slightly better accepted as they were better prepared (Jung et al., 2021, p. 12) though the approach to content was also questioned for various reasons (less flexibility of the online format, fear of open exchange and control under the current political climate). Zoom taught classes mostly worried students in Hong Kong who would not show their faces or speak their mind for privacy concerns and lack of accountability of the platform (Jung et al., 2021, p. 8). As a consequence, more than half disconnected their cameras and felt frustrated by the less interactional and more lecture style format of teaching (Jung et al., 2021, p. 6).

In the UK, it was more a lack of motivation and discouragement due to less direct interaction which led to many students not using their cameras rather than fear of revealing one's identity and privacy concerns as in Hong Kong, although this last point was also an argument put forward by British students.

Even though 26% of Hong Kong students were satisfied by their online learning experience, but similar to the UK, a majority of 60% felt that the learning process was less efficient than face to face (Jung et al., 2021, p. 7). Again, livestream classes appeared new to all students, and even though they were already well familiar with the asynchronous way of sharing documents and PowerPoint before the pandemic, it seems that was even more so the case in Hong Kong where hybrid forms of teaching

---

[3] The Anti-Extradition Law Amendment Bill Movement were a series of demonstrations between 2019 and 2020 in response to the introduction by the Hong Kong government of the Fugitive Offenders amendment bill on extradition. Several of the main universities in Hong Kong were accused of being a stronghold of the movement and violent confrontation between the authorities and protestors who had retreated on university campuses took place, leading to the closing down of campuses and end of teaching activities. (*The New York Times*, 19 November 2019).

and meetings had already been put in place during the phases of political disruption which had preceded the pandemic (Jung et al., 2021, p. 6).

UNESCO's working document on national coping strategies in the education sector did stress that assessment and validation of student learning must be inclusive and fair, accounting for inequalities in access to distance learning facilities (Education Sector, 2020, p. 16). Indeed, students worldwide enjoyed unequal access to technology. In Hong Kong, students unlike teachers were not provided with free cameras and although most are equipped with laptops, some only had a shared home desk computer to work on (Jung et al., 2021, p. 6). It seems that the overall lack of questioning of university support from students may indicate a sense of loss rather than acceptance of their situation (Plakhotnik et al., 2021, p. 10).

6.5 Impact of the Pandemic on the Well-being of Students

Students are considered as a vulnerable group of population for mental health problems because of the transition to adulthood and lack of independent financial means to look after themselves properly (Husky et al., 2020, p. 4). Their mental and economic well-being was therefore affected by the unforeseen circumstances they had to face during the pandemic (loss of student jobs, rent to pay, increasing sense of isolation, and reduced or even lack of social interaction). Several studies including *Covid's Lessons for Global Higher Education: Coping with the Present while Building a More Equitable Future* (Nov. 2020) and the UNESCO report entitled *Covid-19 and Higher education*; *Today and tomorrow: Impact analysis, policy responses and recommendations* (2020) point out the need to examine the ways in which a pandemic may affect staff and students' well-being in order to stem the effects in the future.

Almost two-thirds (63%) of students in the UK indicated that their well-being and mental health had worsened in December since the start of the academic year 2020 (Tinsley, 2020) which is 6% higher than in the previous student survey (20–25 November 2020).

> Over half (56%) of students reported being dissatisfied or very dissatisfied with their social experience since the start of the autumn term. The most common given reasons that students were dissatisfied with their social experience were limited opportunities to meet other students (86%) and limited opportunities for social or recreational activity (85%).

So it would seem that dissatisfaction is widespread as students' current university and private lives do not match their usual expectations. They feel that the pandemic has taken the best of the experience away from them, which explains why so many future students are deferring their bachelor studies hoping for a return to normality or withdrawing from postgraduate studies altogether. For those already enrolled, this new indeterminate situation had an immediate effect on their daily life, cost of living, and other financial burdens as well as the continuation or not of their studies (UNESCO, 15). The crisis confirmed the university as a physical place with students, in particular, missing out on the social experience (European University Association, 4) and all sorts of spontaneous forms of social interactions and support.

In Hong Kong, the purpose of a closed university was questioned as security staff were controlling entry to buildings via the main gates (Jung et al., 2021, p. 7) for the first time in the history of university campuses in Hong Kong. Since early 2020, university campuses went from an open space where anyone could enter for a stroll among the buildings to a closed public space thus announcing a physical change in the city's neighbourhoods. Youth in Hong Kong have a more pessimistic outlook on life in general than the British, especially owing to what they consider as a bleak future in terms of personal freedom because in 2047, Hong Kong will fully reintegrate with China (Jung et al., 2021, p. 5), which is due to the current political tensions which transformed campuses into battling grounds even before the pandemic took place (Lai, 2019) as well as uncertain economic environment. The complete U-turn in the government's position towards masks from banning them in October 2019 to be able to identify protestors in a crowd to cautioning them in February 2020 (Jung et al., 2021, p. 5) also sent a contradictory message to its population which initially contributed to a lasting climate of social confusion and unease. In Hong Kong, face coverings have been mandatory since July 2020 and expanded to outdoor areas in country parks since February 2022 with the arrival of Omicron, which contrasts with the UK when Prime Minister Boris Johnson lifted all the remaining measures in the UK (*Prime Minister's Office*, 21 February 2022).

In the UK, there is no historical landmark to await and more emphasis is laid on a return to normality by all means and the usefulness of wearing a mask was never fully endorsed. Hong Kong's coping strategy seems to have been smoother possibly due to their early acceptance of masks and experience in dealing with pandemics in general.

Masks have been used on public transports for decades in Hong Kong when feeling sick to avoid contaminating others. Indeed, it is considered disrespectful and unpolite not to wear one when you are in a public space if you are likely to contaminate others whereas earlier on in the twentieth century, it would have been perceived as a sign of great sickness. In highly density populated countries, the usefulness of the mask is little questioned especially since the SARS which severely affected China and neighbouring countries in 2002. Asians have grown accustomed to wearing masks for a variety of reasons from air and traffic pollution to dissimulating one's identity with a black face mask as during the Hong Kong protests in 2019 (Jennings, 2020).

In 2020, the OMS had initially reserved the use of a mask for those caring for an infected person until many governments in Europe made them mandatory in public enclosed places and transport. Although legal restrictions have been lifted in the UK since July 2021, the government website still recommends caution and advises individuals to enquire about places and businesses which have chosen to require a mask for their customers. Since January 20 2022, masks are no longer required in classrooms in schools and colleges and from January 27 onwards only recommended on public transport and indoor spaces on the UK government homepage for Coronavirus until they were completely scratched by Prime Minister Boris Johnson on 21 February 2020 (Government UK Homepage, 2022).

Whilst masks seem to be generally better accepted in Asia than in Europe, they remain a sign of environmental and health emergency during a pandemic, for instance. Some staff and advanced students experienced hybrid forms where they were working online from their offices conducting a meeting and wearing a facial covering if with colleagues or fellow students to perform group activities. This could be perceived as a further source of oppression by staff and students during remote work and partial lockdown on top of feeling socially isolated and experiencing pandemic-related anxiety (UNESCO, 2020, p. 15).

6.6 Impact of the Pandemic on Student Work and Career Opportunities

Over the last decade, young people have increasingly been working in occupations that are relatively low paid (Costa Dias, 2020, p. 2) primarily due to an expansion of the accommodation and food industry (Costa Dias, 2020, p. 3). Indeed, these sectors have been shut down during the lockdown which made it harder for young workers to gain some work experience. The economic downturn is also likely to make it harder for workers to progress into higher-paying occupations, which is disrupting early-career wage growth (Costa Dias, 2020, p. 7).The pandemic and policies which followed (lockdown, restrictions) therefore threaten to have a long-term negative economic impact on young people by reducing demand for first timers on the job market and making it harder for young workers to find better alternatives to their current jobs (Costa Dias, 2020, p. 7).

In Hong Kong, where the pandemic struck earlier than in Europe in January 2020, students were also affected but the main difference is that Asian families tend to support students more than in the UK and jobs in unrelated sectors are less crucial to one's career start and development. In Asia, besides connections, building up one's career and network by gravitating in the academic field and obtaining teaching and research contracts pays off in the long run.

According to 2020 figures from major employment platforms, job vacancies in Hong Kong were projected to fall by 55% amidst the economic crisis brought on by the protests and the pandemic (South China Morning Post, 2020). It thus takes longer to get a job and as in the UK, the pay is lower at the start (Jung et al., 2021, p. 9).

Unlike the UK, where many are deferring their undergraduate studies by starting working or going on a gap year (although fluidity of travel is less obvious and job options aboard more limited) while waiting for a permanent return to the normal, there are more applications for Masters degrees as future workers are waiting for the situation to improve and view it more acceptable than being unemployed in the short term (Jung et al., 2021, p. 9). Indeed, there are fewer alternatives and occupations in other sectors but the choice is also made because these options are not as highly regarded and could be perceived as a sign of failure in one's predisposed field. Most Ph.D. graduates in Hong Kong would continue in the academic field (Jung et al.,

2021, p. 10). Competition is fierce, social pressure to succeed is high, and unwavering dedication to one's career path is considered as an essential value. As an illustration, many research papers concerning the impact of the pandemic have been written and educational actors in Hong Kong have remained active throughout the period (Jung et al., 2021, p. 11).

In the UK, one can usually change one's career path more easily and it is commonly held that one's studies are not necessarily immediately applicable to one's work but seen by employers as part of one's background and proof of capacities and skills to develop later on in the workplace.

Project funding which is the basis for Hong Kong graduates to access to a position has been reduced under the new strain. Social economic difference will affect those who can wait for a return to more normal circumstances and those who have to follow a non-academic career path or take an academic position for which they are overqualified (Jung et al., 2021, p. 10). There will be less opportunities to develop one's network in a meaningful way and akin to British students who are stuck in first time low-paid jobs with fewer opportunities to move on to higher-paying ones, graduate students in Hong Kong who mostly move on to academic careers will have less opportunity to do so and may temporarily opt out instead, which makes it even more difficult for them to return to the same field later on.

6.7   Inequalities, Reduced Mobility, and Psychological Impact on Students

Stress occurred most among isolated students rather than those who had been able to relocate home (Husky et al., 2020). There were also some differences between those who live in rural areas and were both more isolated and concerned in case a person close to them had been infected.

Confinement strategies thus have unequal impact on a vulnerable population such as students and may exacerbate social inequalities between those who had options and access to more space like an outdoor garden and those who did not and who were more prone to depression, even if two-thirds of students reported increased stress levels regardless of their location (Husky et al., 2020, p. 7).

Those staying with parents were better off financially (Watermeyer et al., 2021, p. 639) in a context where around 40% of students had to interrupt their jobs or lost them and consequently have been dependent on family support (EUA, 2020, p. 2), with socially disadvantaged students being the least well off.

In the UK, the last year for Erasmus programmes was frozen. In Hong Kong, mobility programmes were also cancelled (Mok et al., 2021, p. 1) and students in China and Hong Kong showed no interest in studying abroad (84%) (Mok et al., 2021, p. 4). Mok et al. (4) wonder if students from Hong Kong will favour universities in nearby Asian countries once the pandemic is over although he notes that the preferred choice is English-speaking universities and especially the US due to employers' interest in innovation and creativity which is what American universities are known for developing. Studying abroad online whilst not travelling and keeping their jobs is at present the preferred choice of many Hong Kong students. There are more options and it is cheaper not to relocate when the quality of digital offering is important, which is a considerable appeal to international students who can pay tuition but not living costs. An influx of new students even if homebased and lower fee-paying could offset the forecasted fall off in international student recruitment which is partly due to the effects of global recession (Watermeyer et al., 2021, p. 639).

6.8 Impact of the Pandemic on Academic Staff

According to a European University Association survey (2013), all institutions offered some amount of online teaching and more than half had planned to develop online degree programmes (EUA, 2020, p. 1). Just before the pandemic started, "most institutions (80%+) indicated that they had in place online repositories for educational materials, a centre or unit that supports teachers on digitally enhanced learning and teaching, as well as digital skills training" (EUA, 2020, p. 1). Most felt ready to teach and assess online at 49.5% though for languages it was down to 30.4%. Confidence was at 60.6% in their ability in doing so (Watermeyer et al., 2021, p. 626) and overall 72.7% felt supported by the institutions in their changing role. (Watermeyer et al., 2021, p. 627).

These figures compare to the level of feeling of dissatisfaction of students (at 37%) who felt unsatisfied by the changed format of education over the same time period (ONS, 2021, p. 4), which shows that over 60% of British students did not really express concerns about the change.

In Hong Kong which operates as a city state, disparity of allocation in resources also exists between disciplines as well as institutions, which were coping as the virus evolved without any long-term strategy (Jung et al., 2021, p. 2). Top universities and scientific sectors like medical and health related which could be seen as contributing to social crisis solving could be viewed positively by society and attracted the most funds (Jung et al., 2021, pp. 11–12). The pandemic has put pressure on academics and publishers to ensure that academic research continues to produce "useful knowledge" (Jung et al., 2021, p. 12).

Even though provisions existed in most universities, it may not have been sufficient for the sudden increased demand, and not all staff and students were familiar with new teaching methods. Provisions and the extent to which communities were prepared also varied from institution to institution. In Hong Kong, cameras were given to staff to teach online, which shows that provisions in terms of equipment were immediate when cautioned by the establishment to keep it functioning properly (Jung et al., 2021, p. 6).

In British universities, staff relied on their own equipment to disseminate knowledge whereas students were able to make loans or borrow equipment when they were barred from using that on site. According to Universities UK (2), the pandemic has deepened inequality between regions in terms of linking skills to students' needs as the higher education system is attracting fewer of those who are less able to select a university that would cater for their learning needs.

The Irish National Digital Experience (INDEX) Survey indicates that 70% of academics in Ireland had never taught online pre-crisis, with similar figures in the UK. Prior to the crisis, academic staff had not been encouraged into making a start with online teaching, as long distance learning courses which were already in place in universities did not rely on face-to-face communication and lecturing. The extent of online teaching was new for unprepared academic staff and it is the suddenness of the switch which revealed weaknesses in usage and delivery. Communication technologies which are already widespread in sectors of society are unanimously regarded as inevitable in the long run to remain in phase with the working world.

However, at the same time, online education was also perceived as disadvantageous to their "occupational welfare" and a "further iteration of neo liberal reform" (Watermeyer et al., 2021, p. 632) and most staff felt reluctant towards fully transitioning to digital education, which they perceive at the same time as dumbing down quality and a cost-saving initiative (Watermeyer et al., 2021, p. 635). The expectation that teachers continue to teach virtually after the end of the pandemic is clearly a source of concern for many (UNESCO, 2020, p. 25), and especially for those who have not been provided with enough tools and adequate training by their institution.

6.9   Assessment of Satisfaction with Content and Delivery by Academic Staff

In the UK, the academic staff felt online teaching had not been satisfactory, but mainly amounted to a didactic transmissional purpose and that they had been fulfilling technical functions and as a consequence, they perceived the whole experience as frustrating and regressive (Watermeyer et al., 2021, p. 631). Posting things online and overuse of technology appeared to be causing role invalidation (Watermeyer et al., 2021, p. 638) and leading to a dumbed down pedagogy associated with the current emergency. For teachers as well as students, higher education had stopped being "a socially immersive experience and participatory learning experience, with the return of the lectern devoid of a larger purpose" (Watermeyer et al., 2021, p. 631). However, the authors remark that online programmes were built under panic and the immense workload of accomplishing this task for the first time without warning put a momentary stress on the work-life balance of individuals and did not contribute to informing on the potential of digital education (Watermeyer et al., 2021, p. 632). In the long term, Watermeyer (632, 638) believes online course curricula could be improved with experience and thus better perceived by purveyors than mere posting of content and interaction as chat discussions. Jung (6) readily admits the advantages of Internet teaching, but he also highlights its limits within the Hong Kong and global contexts.

The prejudice against the dominant use of technology in teaching is still strong especially as the change came suddenly and many teachers fear that their jobs may become obsolete with the shift to online teaching as some institutions like Durham have already moved a quarter of their offer online (Batty, 2020 and Watermeyer et al., 2021, p. 638) and the growing autonomy of students. It is nevertheless mostly teachers on part-time contracts with complementary or practical classes whose jobs have been put at risk by the shift to online modules (UNESCO, 2020, p. 24).

This prejudice may also depend on subjects taught with scientific subjects being more suited to such a format and should be nuanced by the particular circumstances under which change took place. Besides research that directly involved solving the crisis such as working on vaccines and supporting society with related issues has enabled universities to present themselves in a positive light and has enhanced their status. As a consequence, leading universities with health sciences departments are expected to receive more resources and expand their collaborative research with international partners thereby benefiting even further from the crisis (Jung et al., 2021, p. 9).

6.10 Expansive Role of Teaching Staff

The teaching staff felt that they were replacing students support services as tutors to reassure, orientate (Watermeyer et al., 2021, p. 632) and student bodies who were no longer physically present in universities. They felt uneasy and ill prepared in such a counselling role acting as "student support substitutes" (Watermeyer et al., 2021, p. 632). Besides teachers felt such counselling as well as tutoring work from home for long periods of time instead of during regular office hours was inappropriate on top of leading to a blurring of boundaries between work and home life (WHO, 2022). Instead, the tutorial exchanges sounded more like forced group reunions and the online format did not replace all the personal exchanges outside office hours at the beginning and end of seminars, in corridors, lobby areas, cafeteria, and in between seminars. There were as a consequence more time-consuming one-to-one consultations put in place to replace such informal exchanges (Watermeyer et al., 2021, p. 633). Jung insists on the importance of a physical space for students and staff to meet outside class (6) where they would learn and establish some connections.

6.11 Inequality in Career and Advancement

Female academic staff members were less able to publish due to home chores and thus witnessed a slowing down in their career developments with fewer opportunities being offered to them (Watermeyer et al., 2021, p. 633). In Hong Kong, the situation for women was even worse and mothers were most affected when schools stopped for months with online programmes requiring the presence of a parent but also due to caring for elderly relatives (Jung et al., 2021, pp. 7–8). Mothers were more likely to take schooling and care duties in charge thus delaying their career. For instance, one author joked about her daily routine saying she was "a teaching assistant at primary school in the morning and academic at university in the afternoon and evening" (Jung et al., 2021, p. 8).

In Hong Kong, academics were allowed to defer their tenure application by one year to catch up on research and publication and some other adjustments were put in place mostly for women (Jung et al., 2021, p. 8). In the UK, no such measures were taken to support academics whose opportunities were altogether diminished by the pandemic.

6.12   Impact of the Pandemic on the Future Role of Universities

According to Watermeyer, socializing would no longer define university life if personal interaction ends and is replaced by a uniform format, "a product commodified higher education", with fewer faculty members involved. Students would become disengaged from their studies and learning communities (639). In the UK, even if it is not yet the case, abandoning campuses, repurposing halls of residence in central areas, and encouraging the private accommodation sector would certainly affect the local economy, disrupting student areas and businesses which used to cater to them while boosting more residential areas further away from the centre or the historical campuses (Watermeyer et al., 2021, p. 630).

In Hong Kong, institutions are closely connected to their communities by providing recreational spaces for people living in congested urban centres with few parks (O'Sullivan, 2020) and weigh in the attractivity of a neighbourhood. According to Jung (12), "the concept of space in universities has shifted from one that is physically open to society and students and displays strong intellectual dynamism to one that is controlled and empty, and allows for little intellectual engagement". Jung cautions against the loss of informal learning, peer-to-peer exchanges, and cramped living conditions in Hong Kong especially for students unable to study outside libraries (Jung et al., 2021, p. 7).

In both Hong Kong and the UK, new practices in education could make it more diffuse and less connected to a location or body of staff. Students would also face difficulties if their study environment does not facilitate online learning.

A part of the staff felt disorientated especially in the UK, revealing uncomfortable zones (lack of change of institutions) (Watermeyer et al., 2021, p. 624). Some practices were perceived as not in line with labour market requirements and digital transformation deemed insufficient. There was also the fear that teaching would move online whilst reducing overheards (Watermeyer et al., 2021, p. 635) with the non-renewal of fixed-term job contracts. This change was perceived as irreversible (Watermeyer et al., 2021, p. 638). As a consequence of a possible contraction of the higher education sector, more demand would be made on those remaining, despite the lack of homogenous concentration (Watermeyer et al., 2021, p. 639).

Similarly, in Hong Kong, academic staff expected a higher workload and job insecurity following the pandemic (Jung et al., 2021, p. 2) on top of political uncertainty. Since June 2019, anti-government protest had already led to a crisis management so the pandemic was perceived as a way for the education sphere to respond to changes in the environment and find its purpose.

In the UK, the quality of a virtual learning environment may become more appealing than the status and fame of an establishment so the content could represent added value for students which in turn could be positive for universities which are able to adapt to the new post-pandemic requirements (Watermeyer et al., 2021, p. 629). Thus, the quality of online courses may become key to recruiting overseas students in the future. Nevertheless, catching up on technology could remain more uncertain for the less prestigious and less well funded universities which would not attract enough students in a transitory phase. Likewise, in Hong Kong, more competition for online programmes would develop as a result and the most prestigious would be able to withstand competition and resume face-to-face education earlier (Watermeyer et al., 2021, p. 639).

6.13 New Opportunities for Education

According to the European University Association, this may be a historic opportunity to transform learning and teaching (1). The professionalization of education and academics as teachers will lead to a "reinvention of education" (Watermeyer et al., 2021, pp. 636–637). Although all main sources agree that there was some amount of improvisation at the beginning of the pandemic which explains why online migration was not entirely viewed positively (Watermeyer et al., 2021, p. 638), the improvement of the presentation and recordings could offer more control over the lecture and make the experience more inclusive depending on technology and environment (Watermeyer et al., 2021, p. 637). For some academics, they were able to share technological tips and they felt hierarchy had become less important over the period whereas for others, they felt more isolated socially. So at a personal level, the online teaching experience remains contrasted though hybrid options of teaching and doing research are becoming more and more the norm especially when the traditional option has to be put aside (due to manyfold causes such as transport delays, illness, distance). Online interaction limits the disruptions to a programme or activity and enables a smoother functioning of the system, limiting overheads and reducing expenses and commute for off-campus students, for instance.

Research and innovation have been key in the fight against Covid-19, which demonstrated to the wider public the value of expertise and interdisciplinarity. This resulted in increased visibility and appreciation for scientific research. For institutions, research has also been efficient in the move online. Innovative forms of working are being put in place with greater interdisciplinarity and cooperation between centres and external stakeholders (EUA, 2020, p. 5).

For Jung, the new arrangements in the academic field brought benefits for online exchanges and research but they are far from being a solution to all (6). In the medical sector in the UK, students greatly appreciated the flexibility of online teaching platforms but 26.76% felt family distraction was a hindrance and 21.53% blamed a poor Internet connection for slowing down the learning process (Dost et al., 2020). Dost et al. conclude that in the future, online teaching methods will be blended with traditional medical education and that the outcome would be more successful if "medical schools resort to teaching formats such as team-based/problem-based learning", allowing students "to digest information in their own time" but also to discuss this material with peers (Dost et al., 2020., pp. 7–8). This may accompany the observed shift in medical practice towards virtual consultations. Resorting to webinars for foreign short-term visiting academics enabled research to continue to function except for field work and be overall less impacted by the pandemic (Jung et al., 2021, p. 7). Accessibility to seminars has been improved with fewer restrictions on the number of attendees and the removal of physical or geographical barriers whilst tiredness and costs linked to travelling can be eliminated.

6.14   Challenges for Education

On top of mental and physical challenges faced by both universities and students, a clear fall in the number of foreign students notably Chinese students who represent the biggest share in the international market (102,000 as of 2019–20) (Commons Library Briefing, 2021a, p. 3), could be worrying for the stability of the British system. For instance, mainland and Hong Kong Chinese students may be less inclined to travel far at a time when the pandemic is still ongoing and have readapted by studying closer to home in other Asian regions where Chinese is spoken (Mok et al., 2021, pp. 4–5; 8). Although the experience of studying in the UK during a pandemic was rated as bad by 61% of Chinese students who took part in the survey, they may resume their study plans once the pandemic is over (Nott, 2021), which shows that the current trend has not necessarily undermined the long-term popularity of the UK as a study destination.

Decline in international fees will nevertheless continue for a while partly due to a number of recent policies (Commons Library Briefing, 2021a, 2021b, p. 8) and represents a financial hurdle as governments prefer funding social welfare and are globally less committed to education. But while it is clear governments have many competing priorities on their agenda, the enormous benefits generated by universities mean governments should look into providing urgent support (Popov, 2020). Universities generate more than £95 billion for the UK economy and over 940,000 full-time equivalent jobs (Universities UK, 2021, p. 1). Universities need investment from government to protect the student interest, to maintain research capacity, to prevent institutions failing, and to ensure that universities are able to play a central role in the UK's economic and social recovery following the crisis (Universities UK, 2021, p. 1). Universities are playing a leading role in the fight against Covid-19 by supporting local communities and the NHS through research for vaccines and providing thousands of medical and nursing student volunteers and supplying specialist equipment and facilities (Universities UK, 2021, p. 1).

A European Universities Association survey from 2020 (8) points to the prospects of the economy of the European Union shrinking by more than 7%, which is likely to impact, both public and private funding for higher education, and is an additional source of concern. Even though some levelling out of inequalities has taken place (reducing financial costs through online collaborative research projects which could benefit lower-income research students), the difficult economic situation in the UK currently post-Covid could also create unequal opportunities for new graduates. It is less financially secure students who have been most worried about the virus and financially impacted by the non-availability of student jobs during the pandemic.

The possible widening of the gender gap in academia is also apparent. As mentioned before for Hong Kong, female early-career researchers are more vulnerable than their male counterparts. Recent studies have shown that female academics are posting fewer preprints and starting fewer research projects than their male peers, largely because of the increase in teaching tasks during the shift to online teaching and increased childcare responsibilities (King & Frederickson, 2021). Due to family strain and time allocated to online teaching and preparation which requires immediate interaction (online forums, chats, interactive board, etc.), less time may be spent on research by teaching academics, especially women.

In the specific context of Hong Kong, local Ph.D. graduates increasingly face the preference of Hong Kong and mainland Chinese universities for hiring PhDs from universities at the top of world university rankings. Nevertheless, Hong Kong academics are known for their resilience, adaptability to the changing nature of the environment, and capacity to thrive under stress (Jung et al., 2021, p. 12). Regardless of context, students and early-career academics should be better taken into consideration by governments.

It would be interesting to see what the long-term impact of the Covid-19 pandemic will be. How much will virtual exchanges and remote work continue to be used? Will blended learning not only be a remedy in times of social distancing, but a means for more flexible and better quality learning? How will the experience of the crisis help shape collaborative research and promote open access? (EUA, 2020, p. 7) While the university model is often depicted as adverse to change, in the current crisis, it has demonstrated resilience and unforeseen adaptability (EUA, 2020, p. 8). Jung's team questions in their conclusion (12) the definition of knowledge creation in today's higher education and how concepts as well as practices have been challenged during the pandemic.

Governments will have to decide on whether to support the economy, or, to enhance education and health. Funding for research might focus on areas of relevance to Covid-19 while simultaneously lead to fighting for funding in other sectors (de Wit & Altbach, 2021). There might be a loss of student tuition fees in some systems; but in other systems, more people may go to university, to avoid unemployment and prepare for a changed labour market (EUA, 2020, p. 8). Higher education will not become totally virtual. But online teaching and learning as well as online research collaboration and networking will be maintained (de Wit, 2021).

Students and faculty staff are longing to return to campus life and are opting for on campus lectures and exams whenever possible. Academia has proven to be a lively and interactive community that needs to keep an ongoing physical connection. So, finding the right balance between physical and virtual interaction will be key to future developments in the educational field (de Wit, 2021).

References

Ainsworth, S., & Oldfield, J. (2019). Quantifying teacher resilience: Context matters. *Teaching and Teacher Education, 82*, 117–128. https://doi.org/10.1016/j.tate.2019.03.012

Batty, D. (2020, April 17). Lecturers condemn Durham University's plan to shift degrees online. *The Guardian*. https://www.theguardian.com/education/2020/apr/17/lecturers-condemn-durham-universitys-plan-to-shiftdegrees-online

Brazeau, G. A., Frenzel, J. E., & Prescott, W. A. (2020). The Covid-19 pandemic across the academy: Facilitating well-being in a turbulent time. *American Journal of Pharmaceutical Education, 84*(6), 688–691. ncbi.nlm.nih.gov/pmc/articles/PMC7334346/pdf/ajpe8154.pdf

Coron, C., & Dalingwater, L. (Eds.). (2017). *Well-being – Challenging the anglo-saxon hegemony*. Presses Sorbonne Nouvelle.

Chan, Y. K., Kwan, C. C. A., & Shek, T. L. D. (2005). Quality life in Hong Kong: The Cuhk Hong Kong quality of life index. *Social Indicator Research, 71*, 259–289. https://doi.org/10.1007/s11205-004-8020-4

Costa Dias, M., Joyce, R. & Keiller, A. N. (2020, July). *Covid-19 and the career prospects of young people*. Institute for Fiscal Studies Briefing Note BN299. https://ifs.org.uk/uploads/BN299-COVID-19-and-the-career-prospects-of-young-people-1.pdf

de Wit, H. (2021, January 16). *It's getting harder to predict the future of HE*. University World News. https://www.universityworldnews.com/post.php?story=20210115105133419

de Wit, H., & Altbach, P. G. (2021). The post Covid-19 world – Fighting for funding and against inequality post Covid-19. *International Higher Education, 105*. Winter Issue, https://www.internationalhighereducation.net/api-v1/article/!/action/getPdfOfArticle/articleID/3108/productID/29/filename/article-id-3108.pdf

Dost, S., Hossain A., Shehab M., Abdelwahed A., & Al-Nusair L. (2020). Perceptions of medical students towards online teaching during the Covid-19 pandemic: A national cross-sectional survey of 2721 UK medical students. *National Library of Medecine*. https://pubmed.ncbi.nlm.nih.gov/33154063/.

Education Sector. (2020, April). *Covid 19 – A glance of national coping strategies on high-stakes examinations and assessments*. Working Document. Paris: Unesco. https://en.unesco.org/sites/default/files/unesco_review_of_high-stakes_exams_and_assessments_during_covid-19_en.pdf

European University Association. (2020, September). *Briefing – European Higher Education in the Covid-19 crisis*. Brussels: EUA. https://eua.eu/downloads/publications/briefing_european%20higher%20education%20in%20the%20covid-19%20crisis.pdf

Gorge, H., Özçağlar, N., & Toussaint, S. (2015). Bien-être et well-being dans la consommation: une analyse comparative. *Recherche et Applications en Marketing, 30*(2), 104–123. https://doi.org/10.1177/0767370114564137

Government UK Homepage. (2022). www.gov.uk/coronavirus. Last accessed January 2022.

Hamilton, M. (2021, January). *Coronavirus and higher education students: England, 8 January to 18 January 2021*. ONS: Statistical Bulletin. https://www.ons.gov.uk/

peoplepopulationandcommunity/healthandsocialcare/healthandwell-being/bulletins/
coronavirusandhighereducationstudents/8januaryto18january2021

House of Commons Library. (2021a, February 15). *International and EU students in higher education in the UK*. Briefing paper number CBP 7976. www.parliament.uk/commons-library

House of Commons Library. (2021b, February 8). *Coronavirus: Financial impact on higher education*. Briefing paper number 8954. www.parliament.uk/commons-library.

Husky, M. M., Kovess-Masfety, V., & Swendsen, J. D. (2020). Stress and anxiety among university students in France during Covid-19 mandatory confinement. *Comprehensive Psychiatry, 102*, 152191. https://doi.org/10.1016/j.comppsych.2020.152191

Jennings, R. (2020, March 11). Not just coronavirus: Asians have worn face masks for decades. *VOA News*. https://www.voanews.com/science-health/coronavirus-outbreak/not-just-coronavirus-asians-have-worn-face-masks-decades

Jung, J., Horta, H., & Postiglione, G. A. (2021). Living in uncertainty: The Covid-19 pandemic and higher education in Hong Kong. *Studies in Higher Education, 46*(7), 107–120. https://doi.org/10.1080/03075079.2020.1859685

King, M. M., & Frederickson, M. E. (2021). The pandemic penalty: The gendered effects of Covid-19 on scientific productivity. *Socius: Sociological Research for a Dynamic World, 7*, 1–24. https://doi.org/10.1177/23780231211006977

König, A., Graf-Vlachy, L., Bundy, J., & Little, L. M. (2020). A blessing and a curse: How CEOs' trait empathy affects their management of organizational crises. *Academy Management Revolution, 45*, 130–153.

Lai, R. (2019). How universities became the new battle grounds in the Hong Kong protests. *The New York Times*. Last updated November 19, 2019. https://www.nytimes.com/interactive/2019/11/18/world/asia/hong-kong-protest-universities.html

McNamara, A. (2021). Crisis management in higher education in the time of Covid-19: The case of actor training. Special Issue Pedagogic Health and the University. *Education Sciences, 11*(3), 132. https://doi.org/10.3390/educsci11030132

Mok, K. H., Xiong, W., Ke, G., & Cheung, J. O. W. (2021). Impact of Covid-19 pandemic on international higher education and student mobility: Student perspectives from mainland China and Hong Kong. *International Journal of Educational Research, 105*, 101718. https://doi.org/10.1016/j.ijer.2020.101718

Nott W. (2021). Chinese students rate the UK study experience "bad". *The Pie News*. http://thepienews.com/news/uk-61-of-chinese-students-rate-study-experience-as-badduring-pandemic/

O'Sullivan, M. (2020, July 31). *Hong Kong's academics are being isolated in more ways than one*. https://www.timeshighereducation.com/blog/hong-kongs-academics-are-being-isolated-more-ways-one

Pawin, R. (2014). Le bien-être dans les sciences sociales: naissance et développement d'un champ de recherches. *PUF: L'année sociologique 2014/2, 64*, 273–294. https://www.cairn.info/revue-l-annee-sociologique-2014-2-page-273.html

Plakhotnik, M. S., Volkova, N. V., Jiang, C., Yahiaoui, D., Pheiffer, G., Mckay, K., Nerinan, S., & Reissing-Thust, S. (2021). The perceived impact of Covid-19 on student well-being and the mediating role of the university support: Evidence from France, Germany, Russia and the UK. *Frontier Psychology, 12*. https://doi.org/10.3389/fpsyg.2021.642689

Popov, D. (2020, July 14). UK higher education and Covid 19. *Frontier Economics*. http://www.frontier-economics.com/uk/en/news-and-articles/articles/article-i7536-uk-higher-education-and-covid-19

Prime Minister's Office, 10 Downing Street and the Rt Hon Boris Johnson MP (2022 February 21). *PM Statement on living with Covid*. https://www.gov.uk/government/speeches/pm-statement-on-living-with-covid-21-february-2022

Salmi, J. (2020, November). *Covid's lessons for global higher education. Coping with the present whilst building a more equitable future*. Indianapolis, IL: Lumina Foundation. https://www.

luminafoundation.org/wp-content/uploads/2020/11/covids-lessons-for-global-higher-education.pdf

South China Morning Post. (2020, May 18). *Tough ride ahead for Hong Kong graduates, as job vacancies fall 55 per cent amid economy battered by protests, pandemic employment prospect.* https://www.scmp.com/news/hong-kong/education/article/3084768/tough-ride-ahead-hong-kong-graduates-job-vacancies-fall-55.

Tay, L. (2021). Building community well-being in higher education: An introduction to the special issue. *International Journal of Community Well-being, 4,* 461–466. https://doi.org/10.1007/s42413-021-00144-4

Tinsley, B. (2020). *Coronavirus impact on students in Higher Education in England: September to December 2020.* https://www.ons.gov.uk/peoplepopulationandcommunity/education andchildrenarticles/coronavirusandtheimampactonstudentsinhighereducationinEngland SeptembertoDecember2020/2020-12-21

UNESCO. (2020). *COVID-19 and higher education: Today and tomorrow; Impact analysis, policy responses and recommendations.* Institut international de l'UNESCO pour l'enseignement supérieur en Amérique latine et dans les Caraïbes. https://unesdoc.unesco.org/ark:/48223/pf0000375693

Universities UK. (2021). *Achieving stability in the higher education sector following Covid-19 - A proposal to government for a balanced package of measures to maximise universities' contribution to the economy, communities and the post virus recovery.* https://www.universitiesuk.ac.uk/what-we-do/policy-and-research/publications/achieving-stability-uk-higher-education

Veenhoven, R., & Brulé, G. (2014). Average happiness and dominant family type in regions in Western Europe around 2000. *Advances in Applied Sociology, 4*(12), 271–288. https://doi.org/10.4236/aasoci.2014.412031

Wales P. (2021, March 31). *Coronavirus and the impact on measures of UK government education output: March 2020 to February 2021.* ONS Government UK. https://www.ons.gov.uk/economy/grossdomesticproductgdp/articles/coronavirusandtheimpactonmeasuresofuk governmenteducationoutput/march2020tofebruary2021

Watermeyer, R., Crick, T., Knight, C., & Goodall, J. (2021). Covid-19 and digital disruption in UK universities: Afflictions and affordances of emergency online migration. *Higher Education, 81,* 623–641. https://doi.org/10.1007/s10734-020-00561-y

Whitehall Well-being Working Group. (2006). *Well-being: Statement of common understanding,* Working Paper.

WHO (2022, February 2). *WHO says working from home creates blurring of boundaries.* https://www.openaccessgovernment.org/who-working-from-home/128758/

Wong, M. Y. S., Siu, L. T. T., Hui, L. M. C. H., Chan, K. W. S., Lee, H. M. E. & Chang, W. C. (2021). Changes in mental well-being in Hong Kong before and during social unrest and Covid-19. https://doi.org/10.21203/rs.3.rs-440216/v1

Iside Costantini is an associate professor in British Politics/Civilization at the Sorbonne Nouvelle University, Paris. She completed a Ph.D. in 2009 on nineteenth century exchanges between Great Britain and South China (Hong Kong, Canton, Shanghai) through the English-language press. She has developed an interest for Sino-British relations from the nineteenth to the twenty-first centuries including comparative approaches in well-being policies/issues. She contributed a chapter "Confucianism Promoted as an Alternative to the Anglo-Saxon Social-Cultural Model" in *Well-being—Challenging the Anglo-Saxon Hegemony* (Presses Sorbonne Nouvelle, 2017) and coedited an online volume *Well-being: Political Discourse and Policy in the Anglosphere* (Papers in Political Economy, 2019).

Chapter 7
Mental Health and Well-being During Covid-19 Forced Distance Learning Period: Good and Bad News from Polish Studies

Jacek Pyżalski and Natalia Walter

Abstract The chapter focuses on empirical findings from significant Polish studies conducted during different phases of the pandemic (mostly quantitative surveys on teacher and student samples, but qualitative aspects will also be included). Among those presented, we will use data from a large project carried out in 34 schools where students (N = 1284), teachers (N = 671), and parents (N = 979) were surveyed in May and June 2020 (Ptaszek et al., Edukacja zdalna: co stało się z uczniami, ich rodzicami i nauczycielami?, Gdańskie Wydawnictwo Psychologiczne, 2020). Apart from this, we present and interpret data from other, sometimes smaller scale projects using both a quantitative and qualitative approach. Structurally, it will cover the issues of mental health and well-being of young people (health self-assessment, depression, psychosomatic complaints) as well as the factors influencing those variables (quality of peer relations, family relations, quality of ICT usage). Furthermore, the selected data on the health and well-being of important adults (teachers and parents) will be presented, as their state should be analysed as connected to the well-being of young people.

Conceptually, we will also extract the groups of young people particularly sensitive and experiencing problems during the pandemic, such as young people with special needs and their siblings, young people experiencing negative home situations, etc. We will present this group as one that deserves particular help and support. We will also present the results showing that there is a small but significant group of young people that during the pandemic had the opportunity to experience numerous positive events and had a positive impact on their functioning and development. The chapter concludes with selected ideas concerning both the distance education time during the pandemic and the organization of educational and support systems in the period of return of young people to educational institutions.

J. Pyżalski · N. Walter (✉)
Adam Mickiewicz University, Poznan, Poland
e-mail: Natalia.Walter@amu.edu.pl

© The Author(s), under exclusive license to Springer Nature Switzerland AG 2022
L. Dalingwater et al. (eds.), *The Unequal Costs of Covid-19 on Well-being in Europe*,
Human Well-Being Research and Policy Making,
https://doi.org/10.1007/978-3-031-14425-7_7

7.1 Young People and Mental Health During the Crisis: Introductory Remarks

The period of remote education during the Covid-19 pandemic has been called a crisis or forced remote education in the scientific literature that describes different psychosocial aspects of that period (Bozkurt & Sharma, 2020; Murphy, 2020; Pyżalski, 2020). Those terms clearly underline the specific character of our experiences. Firstly, the educational system was not sufficiently prepared (both in Poland and other countries, including those with longer traditions in remote education) to conduct remote education in a way that fully meets the needs of the children (Doucet et al., 2020; United Nations, 2020). Secondly, this period meant changes and problems in other, not so obvious areas. Among them, it is worth mentioning such issues as relationships vital for education (mainly peer and teacher–student relationships), factors related to the well-being and mental health of students and teachers, as well as digital well-being related (connected to qualitative and quantitative shifts in the use of information and communication technologies).

For contextual information, one has to mention that Poland was the country that with some exceptions (as selected special education institutions) has maintained remote education in the years 2020 and 2021 for the longest time compared to other European countries. It lasted from 13 months of actual remote lessons to even more in some schools where the pandemic situation has been worse.

Since our text is based on empirical studies, it is worth mentioning some methodological aspects of social science research that substantially impact the quality of the research material gathered and the conclusions drawn from it.

On the one hand, that time was "a golden era" for social science researchers. There were numerous issues that could have been and that actually had been explored. However, certain aspects of research processes complicated the life of researchers and significantly impacted research procedures. An important thing was the difficulty in getting in touch with the research population. The only possibility left in place of traditional contacts was the Internet-mediated contact. Unfortunately, the latter are also impacted by digital inequalities in their basic understanding, namely, lack of hardware or Internet connection. That simply means that when conducting research online, we systematically use this excluded group of young people and adults from the research samples. The result was that we learnt almost nothing about those groups that are potentially highly impacted. The mode of collection of material also impacted the quality of the samples. Many scholars decided to ask respondents to participate through links to social networking sites. That is a tempting method allowing us to easily complete large samples. However, those samples of volunteers are substantially different from general populations, so the results obtained cannot be extrapolated to them. Additionally, online versions of the research instrument have different psychometric properties from traditional versions. On top of this, the Covid-19 pandemic was a dynamic process, which means that all psychological and social processes change in time and have different consequences. That means that even the difference in weeks or months in data collection points may be significant for interpretation of the results. All of this, of course, does not mean that the research data from the time of crisis remote education are irrelevant. Still, it is vital to be extremely cautious and critical, particularly when studies are followed by practical conclusions and their interpretation. Additionally, in many cases, there were no longitudinal data to compare the results from the remote education period to the time before the pandemic.

It is also worth noting that although this period is commonly viewed as a threat to the mental health of children and adults, there is also a certain proportion of the population who have benefited from changes in psychosocial circumstances.

In this chapter, we focus mainly on the results of research from our country— Poland). Predominantly, we present the data from a large project carried out in 34 schools where students (N = 1284), teachers (N = 671), and parents (N = 979) were surveyed in May and June 2020 (zdalnenauczanie.org) (Ptaszek et al., 2020). Yet, we refer partially to literature from other countries to add more context and opportunities for comparison.

7.2 Self-assessment of General Health Status and Quality of Life

Mental health issues became crucial during the pandemic and attracted the attention and efforts of mental health and educational professionals (both researchers and practitioners). At the same time, much less attention was paid to the health of adults, namely, parents/guardians and teachers, within the context of this text. Our approach to this issue is holistic. We acknowledge that the mental health of young people and important adults (mainly parents and teachers) in their environment is interrelated.

Focusing on mental health should not be surprising since the time of the pandemic and e-learning is very rich in risk factors which, at least for some people, could and, as research shows, have caused a number of negative consequences in this area.

The results of a large-scale study on teenagers, their parents, and teachers, conducted in Poland entitled "Remote learning and adaptation to social conditions during the coronavirus epidemic" (Ptaszek et al., 2020) confirmed that in all those groups there was a significant proportion of those who felt their mental health decreased during the pandemic. However, among those three groups, the proportion of students who felt much worse or slightly worse was the lowest (18% felt a lot worse and 30% slightly worse). These results were also related to age, with a higher proportion of older students experiencing this deterioration. It is also worth noting that around 50% of young people observed severe mild negative changes in their physical health (Bigaj & Dębski, 2020). As in the holistic approach, physical and mental health should be understood as "two sides of the same coin", this result is also of great importance when evaluating the health status of young people during the Covid pandemic.

These results are in line with those of another study on life satisfaction among young people during the pandemic. About a third of young people, aged 13–17, assessed their level of satisfaction with life poorly. The same proportion stated that their well-being compared to the time before the school closure had deteriorated. All these negative symptoms were higher in girls (Makaruk et al., 2020).

There were more individuals who felt worse mentally among parents (14%—a lot worse and 40%—worse). The highest percentage has been observed in the teacher group (30% and 35%, respectively). Another study, conducted seven months after school closure in Poland, showed that a significant proportion of teachers was found to have high scores indicating mental health difficulties—16% high or moderately high scores on depression symptoms, and 29% high scores on general anxiety (Pisula et al., 2020). The latter results are particularly important as the mental health of students is also largely determined by the health and well-being of important adults around them. In this context, a question may be asked whether, for example, it is possible for a teacher whose mental state has deteriorated to be able to effectively support the mental health of students.

To conclude, the results confirm that during the remote crisis education period, both young people and adults felt worse. It was particularly supported by analysing those research data where respondents compared their state during school closure to the period before. This is surely an important result but not sufficient from a practical perspective—here we need a more detailed picture of mental health problems during school closure and the important factors that influence them. The broader perspective of observing not only the mental health of young people, but also that of adults, has also brought another dimension worth considering. This is connected to the fundamental question whether adults affected negatively themselves by the pandemic period can successfully support the mental health of the younger generation? Of course, this question is rather rhetorical, and it should be understood rather as an appeal to support the mental health of teachers. Finally, this positively impacts the quality of work of teachers and their ability to support the mental health of young people. This is a valid issue not only for the time of the pandemic, but also in the transition time from remote to traditional education in physical places. This time is rich with numerous challenges to the mental health of young people. Therefore, they need the teachers to support them in this process. Again, if educational professionals struggle with their own mental health, they can experience difficulties in providing high-quality communication and support to young people.

7.3 Depression and Mood Disorders

Depression and mood disorders have been diagnosed as a serious issue in the young population also before the pandemic (e.g. Ostaszewski et al., 2005; Ryan, 2005). They are frequently connected with the most serious consequences including suicidal ideation. During the pandemic, depression and mood disorders have been frequently explored by researchers, as it was assumed that they may increase due to the specific determinants present during that period. Most of the studies confirmed this prediction. During remote crisis education, a high level of depressive moods has been observed in 23% of girls and 8% of boys in Polish schools. Girls had more frequent symptoms such as sadness, loneliness, depression, or desire to cry all time. Furthermore, symptoms of negative mood disorders were more frequent among older respondents (Pisula et al., 2020).

Such problems were also present in adults. A significant proportion of teachers indicated high scores on mental health difficulties—16% high or moderately high scores on depression symptoms and 29% high scores on experiencing anxiety (Pisula et al., 2020). Other studies prove an even more serious situation (Bigaj & Dębski, 2020).

About one in ten surveyed Polish adolescents indicated certain symptoms of depressive mood: 9% of them felt sad all the time, 10% were lonely all time, and felt depressed. Severe symptoms of depression (based on the frequency) concerned 17% of teachers, 13% of parents, and 5% of students (Bigaj & Dębski, 2020).

A similar picture emerges from the analysis of the opinions of school staff on the needs of young people regarding mental health. The results of the survey conducted by Fundacja Szkoła z Klasą (2021) indicate depression as the most serious problem—it was mentioned by 40% of the surveyed teachers. According to the self-reports of the above-mentioned students, teachers perceived depression more often as a problem of older students (Fundacja Szkoła & Klasą, 2021).

7.3.1 Depression and Mood Disorders Are Frequently Associated with Psychosomatic Symptoms

Studies conducted during school closure generally confirm a high prevalence of psychosomatic complaints among young people. A significant proportion of adolescents experienced psychosomatic problems. In the older adolescents' group, sleep disturbances during the 30 days preceding the study occurred at least once in 60% of the respondents (in 22% several times or more). A significant percentage of young people often (more than a dozen times a month) suffered headaches (16%) or abdominal pain (9%). In turn, more than one in three experienced a lack of energy (Bigaj & Dębski, 2020). Other results also confirm the frequent appearance of psychosomatic problems in young people in secondary schools during school closure (Długosz, 2020).

In conclusion, depressive symptoms were observed more often during the pandemic in both young people and adults compared to the situation before school closure (Ostaszewski et al., 2005). However, the rise is not as substantial as sometimes presented by the media. However, preventive measures (including early detection) were crucial during the pandemic and after returning to school buildings. Particularly important here is the possibility that mood disorders and depression have been found during the pandemic, the experience of other young people than before. That requires a lot of attention and willingness from school personnel to help, as well as to seek professional psychological/psychiatric treatment in more serious cases.

Again, the results concerning teachers are particularly important as the mental health of students is to a large extent determined by the health and well-being of education professionals (Harding et al., 2019). It is doubtful that teachers experiencing serious mood disorders are able to maintain proper relationships with their students and support their mental health.

7.4 Important Factors Influencing the Mental Health of Young People

For analytical purposes in this chapter, we present not only the mental health consequences but also factors that were present during the school closure and influence health and well-being during this time. It is worth underlying that factors such as digital well-being or the quality of important relationships can also be treated as indicators of mental health itself. Moreover, since they are more flexible and easier to change, it is more rational to understand them as influencing factors. This is particularly valid when we take a practical approach focusing on the environmental changes that may be implemented. Knowledge on those factors may also be a basis for proper integration programmes that should be implemented while shifting from remote to traditional education.

7.4.1 Digital Well-being

Research shows that nowadays we are almost constantly online. Smartphones are constantly touched and are for the young generation the main tool for being online (Deng et al., 2019; Dscout, 2016; Pyżalski et al., 2019; Sewall et al., 2020). The newest EU Kids Online report indicates that the amount of time spent online by young people has almost doubled in all countries participating in the study compared to the same study results from 2010 (Smahel et al., 2020). During the pandemic, the time spent online on both school days and weekends doubled (Bigaj & Dębski, 2020). For sure, time itself is not a sufficient indicator of a potential negative influence on mental health. This is particularly true with mobile Internet and various modes of using it—e.g. there is a big difference between using online navigation while running and playing a game on a smartphone screen.

Smartphone use (or rather mobile Internet use) proved to distract from work and study (Duke & Montag, 2017; Rosen et al., 2013), leading to procrastination (Schnauber-Stockmann et al., 2018), sleep disturbances (Gustafsson et al., 2017; Lanaj et al., 2014), or evoked negative emotions such as emotional exhaustion

(Büchi et al., 2019). Earlier scientific evidence has also indicated that screen time is associated with obesity, hypertension, type 2 diabetes, myopia, depression, sleep disturbance, and other health conditions. This increased burden of disease is more common among sedentary people and applies to children, adolescents, and teachers who spend many hours a day using computers or smartphones during online lessons.

On the positive side of this, we have digital well-being understood as a subjective, individual experience of the optimal balance between the benefits and disadvantages of using mobile screen media. This empirical state comprises affective and cognitive assessments of the integration of digital connectivity with ordinary life. People achieve digital well-being when they experience maximum controlled pleasure and functional support, with minimal loss of control and functional impairment while using new media (Vanden Abeele, 2020).

Disturbed digital well-being may also lead to problematic Internet use as another side of the continuum. The latter is understood as the collection of negative symptoms present when the Internet is used in an unhealthy way (e.g. overwhelming all other activities, influencing negative school engagement, etc.) (Makaruk et al., 2019). This issue was also examined by researchers who analysed the situation of students and teachers during a remote educational crisis around the world (Sultana et al., 2021). The study by Ptaszek et al. (2020) shows that 66% of the students admitted that they often or very often use screen tools just before going to sleep, and half of them (50%) said that they felt overwhelmed with information. Over half of the teachers and some students felt very often or often snoozed due to the use of the Internet, a computer, or a smartphone. More than a quarter of students very often or often during online classes used smartphones, social networking sites, played games, browsed the Internet for private purposes, or wrote to someone unrelated to the lessons.

It is astonishing that the same problems attributed usually to students also appear in teachers, sometimes even in a higher proportion. More than 85% of teachers declared that they were often or very often constantly ready to receive calls and notifications, or that they were often or very often tired of sitting at the computer. Three-quarters felt tired and overloaded with information present in the media. The extended screen time during the Covid-19 pandemic has become the subject of numerous studies around the world (e.g. Colley et al., 2020; Sikorska et al., 2021; Sultana et al., 2021).

The available evidence shows that digital well-being should have been the centre of mental health support for young people during school closures and is still a major concern. Therefore, evidence-based interventions should be implemented to prevent the consequences of deteriorated digital well-being and to teach and support the constructive and healthy use of new media. They can, among other things, promote an active lifestyle and participation in outdoor activities (Oberle et al., 2020; Sultana et al., 2021). It is also clearly seen that problems with digital well-being are also experienced by adults. This brings attention to the potential negative role modelling as well as the necessity to avoid the implementation of programmes assuming that such problems are only on the side of young people.

7.4.2   Decreasing the Quality of Important Relations (Peer, Student–Teacher)

The mental health issues discussed previously are directly related to the quality of educationally important relationships and what happened to them at the time of school closure. Surprisingly, the interest of researchers and the public in these issues was relatively small at the beginning. It only attracted attention and was discussed in the media just before returning to educational institutions.

The relationships are based on communication that turned from the traditional mode to the so-called computer-mediated one (Romiszowski & Mason, 1986). Therefore, initially, the analysis involved key technical issues (what hardware and software to use and how) and later organizational and conceptual aspects (what is important in building relationships based on online contacts? How to use them from an educational perspective?). In the first practical crisis remote education guide published in Poland—"Education in the times of the Covid-19 pandemic. With a distance from what we are currently doing as teachers", the need to treat relations in remote education as a priority and constitute the necessary foundation for didactic activities was clearly advised (Pyżalski & Poleszak, 2020). The reason for such an approach is also the common experience of communicational difficulties that teachers often explained. They often indicate the limitations of the contact possibilities available when we communicate in an indirect way (such as the number of people who can be seen simultaneously on the screen while conducting a synchronous remote lesson).

The perspective of the students was similar. The qualitative part of a large Polish study, conducted in 34 schools in May and June 2020, with a sample of older teenagers, showed that the surveyed students missed their peer relationships the most (Stunża, 2020). In the quantitative part of the same research, 50% of the students surveyed indicated that their relations with their classmates before the pandemic were much or slightly better. At the same time, 39% of the respondents did not notice any changes in this area (Pyżalski, 2020a). It is worth noting that although the percentage of young people indicating a deterioration in peer relations is significant, it is far from being such that it would justify generalizations indicating that the majority of the young population assess the quality of peer and student–teacher relations as worse.

In conclusion, relationships based on online communication tend to deteriorate according to a significant proportion of young people. However, similar percentages of young respondents claimed that they did not notice any changes in the quality of the relationships or even perceived them as improved. Based on this, one should analyse what makes maintaining high-quality relations with some young people possible, while others perceive them as weaker. This knowledge is important for designing and implementing educational and support activities in case of possible repetition of distance education need in the future (due to a pandemic or other reasons) (Walter, 2020). Research results also show the need to pay significant attention to activities that support peer and student–teacher relationships after return.

7.5   Who Was at the Highest Risk?

In many cases, particularly in media representations, the risk of mental health for young people during remote crisis education was presented as the same level for the entire population of young people. Therefore, there were many discussions where specialists presented potential areas of harm caused by factors present during the pandemic. However, adopting such an approach may cause us to fail to recognize that there are differences among the groups of young people regarding the potential effects of the pandemic period. Additionally, there are groups that are more vulnerable than others and need special support both during the pandemic and after returning. Below, we look closer and analyse the situation of such subgroups.

7.5.1   Digitally Excluded Due to Lack of Technology

One of the fundamental issues related to remote crisis education during the pandemic was access to tools for conducting and participating in distance learning, both for students and teachers. Such access is clearly a prerequisite for educational and social activities that should be possible in times where computer-mediated communication is only possible (Gajderowicz & Jakubowski, 2020).

Centrum Cyfrowe research from the first period of the pandemic, conducted in April 2020 (Buchner et al., 2020) (just after school closure) showed that 36% of teachers considered the main problem during remote education as deficiencies in student equipment, and for 51% it was problematic to overcome it. It was caused primarily by the fact that parents working remotely used household equipment that their children could previously use. It has become impossible for all family members to share equipment at the same time. Families with many children or in a difficult financial situation had great difficulties in this respect. Similarly, regarding students' Internet connections: it was the main problem for 32% of teachers and a problem that could be solved for 56%. The hardware deficiencies of the teachers themselves were the main problem for 10%, while 46% have coped with this issue effectively. In the second edition of the Centrum Cyfrowe research (Buchner & Wierzbicka, 2020) conducted in the fall of 2020, the shortcomings of students' equipment became a slightly smaller challenge, although it was still the main problem for one-third of teachers.

In extreme cases, the exclusion of students from remote education was complete. They simply disappeared from the classroom, and teachers often had serious difficulties contacting the students and their parents or guardians. Unfortunately, these issues were not systematically diagnosed, let alone solved in our country. However, some studies conducted indicate the scale of such problems. An example of the diagnosis shown by this is the second report of Centrum Cyfrowe, where up to 48% of teachers in primary and secondary schools indicated that at least one of their students had disappeared. This percentage was higher among professional school teachers and reached 58% (Buchner & Wierzbicka, 2020).

Although digital exclusion due to lack or insufficient access to technology (digital tools and Internet connection) seems to be a thing of the past, the pandemic period has shown that it is still a problem. As without such access, all online activities provided by educational institutions are impossible, it is crucial for the national system to monitor and address inequalities in this area.

7.5.2 Young People with Special Needs

The key group that experienced inequality in the period of interest to us was young people with special educational needs (Plichta, 2020; Plichta et al., 2020). The hardest challenge was to adapt the lessons to the needs of people with disabilities (particularly sensory ones). Numerous applications that enable synchronous communication do not fully take into account the special educational needs of students. There were difficulties inviting sign language interpreters to the lessons and displaying it clearly on the screen along with the image of the teacher and his activities, e.g., on the blackboard. Many teachers used visual elements during lessons that were useful for well-sighted people, while for those with sight impairments, they were a great difficulty and brought many limitations.

Empirical analyses in this area were carried out by a team led by Ewa Domagała-Zyśk (2020). During the distance education of the pandemic, young people and children with special educational needs experienced many burdensome situations, including those related to access to the IT infrastructure and the quality of relationships with teachers and other students. Experiencing difficulties resulting from a specific disability was a particular burden for them. An example may be young people with hearing disabilities who experience numerous communication problems related to the use of indirect communication by teachers (which was often not adapted to their needs). The consequence was negative emotions related to difficulties in full participation in educational activities (Lewandowska, 2020). Many students with special needs (for example, those with intellectual disabilities, students on the autism spectrum who had difficult access to therapy during their education) experienced an increase in difficult behaviours (Kułaga, 2020). In this context, remote education has added special challenges related to individualization of interactions and meeting special educational needs.

Another group that experienced problems related to remote education in a particularly negative way were young people staying in care and educational institutions of various types. Qualitative research conducted in these institutions identified a number of important problems related to distance education during a pandemic in this type of institution (Ruszkowska, 2020). Hardware problems were an essential issue here. There is rarely enough equipment and good quality Internet connection that is sufficient for students to use it when required. This often translated into the inability to participate in online classes. The challenges related to the organization of educational support were even greater. The educators were unable to effectively support the students (often experiencing severe learning difficulties) in all subjects. Furthermore, due to the pandemic time, these institutions, both in terms of didactic and educational issues, were deprived of volunteer support for epidemiological reasons.

7.5.3 Children Victimized at Home

Particularly vulnerable and at risk of serious mental health problems is the group of young people who experienced victimization at home or at least perceived communication with adult family members as much worse during school closure. About 13% of young people admitted that their relationships with their parents or guardians deteriorated (Pyżalski, 2020a). Furthermore, up to 17% indicated more frequent quarrels with household members (Pyżalski, 2020b). Unfortunately, this was often accompanied by a decline in activities important for family life, such as conversations with family members (11%) or help with household chores (11%) (Pyżalski, 2020b).

The scale and importance of the problems of this group are confirmed by the research of the Empowering Children Foundation, which indicates that approximately one in nine teenagers experienced violence from their relatives during the pandemic, most often from family members (Makaruk et al., 2020). Such violence (mainly verbal) was more common among older teenagers and people living in rural areas. Five percent of teenagers have also witnessed domestic violence against another child or adult (Makaruk et al., 2020).

The biggest challenge in this context was to provide early detection of such problems during the pandemic as well as to provide professional help both during remote education and after returning. The specific problem may here result in "masking" those negative experiences after return by reactions that are difficult for teachers to interpret and cope with (e.g. rude behaviour).

The groups experienced positive effects during the pandemic circumstances. Although the period of remote education of crisis is commonly interpreted as the time that brought threats and worsened the state of mental health of the young population, there is a certain proportion of young people who experienced this time as empowering. or instant in the Polish study, one in six students indicated that they felt a little or much better during school closure (9% and 8%, respectively) (Bigaj & Dębski, 2020).

The same was true for the important factors that positively influence mental health. For example, as shown by longitudinal studies by psychologists from the University of Warsaw, many parents and students indicated an improvement in home relationships related to specific activities of parents and children (Gambin et al., 2020).

There was a special group of students among whom the positive changes during the pandemic were spectacular. The analysis of the content of the interviews with teachers shows that they notice students who, during the closure of schools, gained many benefits in the area of learning quality, relationships with other people (teacher and peers), etc. The examples indicated by teachers allow us to indicate the following groups of students, some of whom, according to the teachers, have benefited from the pandemic. Below, we introduce the main groups of this kind and short descriptions.

7.5.4 Students Experiencing Difficulties in Public Communication

In many cases, remote communication (e.g. speaking without a camera) made these students feel safer and gave them the courage to speak. This was mainly due to the fact that public appearances evoked less intensity of emotion in them, which previously blocked them. In many cases, teachers indicated that they had heard the statements of some students during remote education for the first time, even though they had worked with these students for a long time.

7.5.5 Peer Violence Victims

During remote education, students were less accessible to the aggressors, they did not spend much time with them. Thus, they were less likely to be victims of bullying. For this group, the pandemic period was a good time not to experience unpleasant and hostile situations and sometimes even to link positively with their peers (mostly using online communication).

7.5.6 Students with Special Educational Needs, For Example, Autism Spectrum Disorder

It should be noted that, as stated above, for most students with special educational needs, this period was a serious risk to their mental health. However, we should notice that some students had the opportunity to avoid stimuli that previously distracted them during classroom learning (e.g. noise). They also had greater opportunities to work in an individualized way (e.g. at their own pace).

7.5.7   Students with a Fixed Negative Position/Image in the Group

Many students who functioned with an established stereotypical image in the classroom (e.g. the image of "someone who does not care about learning") during remote education, when they ceased to be so visible to other students, found themselves in a situation where they could comfortably start functioning differently (e.g. engaging more in classroom activities).

For some of those students, mediated communication made it possible to benefit from teacher support without having to attract the attention of the whole group (e.g. in a private chat). In many cases, these students received support (e.g. in the form of individual explanations of difficult issues), which allowed them to make progress.

The results and analysis presented above show that the pandemic period is unjustly treated as having only a negative impact on the mental and physical health of young people. There is a significant proportion (although it is clearly a minority) of those who, based on different reasons, benefited from this time and improved their mental health and, in many cases, social competence. Paradoxically, for this group, at least in some cases, returning to traditional education may be a risk. Some of those students, while deprived of factors specific to the time of school closure, may suddenly lose all the benefits they had during this time. They may be associated with negative emotions and frustration. From this perspective, the group of those who benefitted can be understood as a group with a high risk of mental health problems after returning to traditional education.

7.6   Conclusions

When we analyse the period of the forced remote period, it seems obvious that it was the time of an unprecedented negative influence on the mental health of both adults and young people. Two types of negative factors seem to bring the highest risk. The first one is a substantial negative change of the way people communicate and subsequently the quality of important interpersonal relations. These main relations are, in an educational context student–teacher relations and peer relations. The second potential risk factor is the technology itself or rather the way technology is used (e.g. problematic Internet use).

Research results on those factors may also, at least partially, provide answers to the question about how one can support the mental health of young people both during the time of the pandemic or similar or after return. First, one should focus on exploring the possibility of initiating and maintaining important educational relations based on communication mediated by new technologies (Walter & Pyzalski, 2022). They provide numerous opportunities to experience contacts and relations that are real, although they require specific competencies and attitudes on the side of teachers and students. This may be also used in the long term also after the pandemic when technology is used as a choice by educators and students but not a necessity. Additionally, as relations have deteriorated (as assessed by quite high proportions of students) it is important to focus on peer relationships after returning to school. This means implementing measures aimed at connecting students and providing numerous opportunities and time for communication.

Digital well-being should also be addressed but not only understood narrowly as a problem of the young generation, but holistically as something that is crucial for young people and adults. The available guidelines should be reviewed and evidence-based interventions should be considered to prevent the effects of the deterioration of digital well-being after the pandemic period, also by promoting offline activities such as physical activity.

The most important thing is also adopting a perspective that acknowledges the differences between young people and adults regarding the potential negative influence of the distance education period. That also means defining specific groups that are significantly more vulnerable and addressing them with special programmes that support mental health. From this perspective, the crucial thing is the mental health of teachers since they should have the potential to support children and adolescents. Unfortunately, such potential is significantly impaired when adults suffer themselves (Brockman et al. 2019; Pyżalski & Merecz, 2010).

Lastly, we should also observe that for some subgroups of young people, the specificity of Covid-19 remote education period brought a lot of benefits and adults (particularly the teaching staff) should take heed so that they do not just disappear just after a return to traditional classroom learning, e.g. to take measures that the students who started to be verbally active during remote education lessons do not withdraw again on return to school.

References

Bigaj, M., & Dębski, M. (2020). Subiektywny dobrostan i higiena cyfrowa w czasie edukacji zdalnej. In G. Ptaszek, G. D. Stunża, J. Pyżalski, M. Dębski, & M. Bigaj (Eds.), *Edukacja zdalna: co stało się z uczniami ich rodzicami i nauczycielami?* GWP.

Bozkurt, A., & Sharma, R. C. (2020). Emergency remote teaching in a time of global crisis due to Corona Virus pandemic. *Asian Journal of Distance Education, 15*(1), i–vi.

Brockman, R., Campbell, R., Araya, R., Murphy, S., & Kidger, J. (2019). Is teachers' mental health and well-being associated with students' mental health and well-being? *Journal of Affective Disorders, 253*, 460–446.

Büchi, M., Festic, N., & Latzer, M. (2019). Digital overuse and subjective well-being in a digitized society. *Social Media+Society., 5*(4). https://doi.org/10.1177/2056305119886031

Buchner, A., Majchrzak, M., & Wierzbicka, M. (2020). *Edukacja zdalna w czasie pandemii.* Raport. Edycja I. Warszawa: Fundacja Centrum Cyfrowe. https://centrumcyfrowe.pl/edukacja-zdalna/

Buchner, A. & Wierzbicka, M. (2020). *Edukacja zdalna w czasie pandemii.* Raport. Edycja II. Warszawa: Fundacja Centrum Cyfrowe. https://centrumcyfrowe.pl/edukacja-zdalna/

Colley, R., Bushnik, T., & Langlois, K. (2020). Exercise and screen tine during the COVID-19 pandemic. *Statistics Canada—Health Reports, 31*(6), 3–11. https://doi.org/10.25318/82-003-x202000600001-eng

Deng, T., Kanthawala, S., Meng, J., Peng, W., Kononova, A., Hao, Q., et al. (2019). Measuring smartphone usage and task switching with log tracking and self-reports. *Mobile Media & Communication, 7*(1), 3–23. https://doi.org/10.1177/2050157918761491

Długosz, P. (2020). *Raport z badań: „Krakowska młodzież w warunkach kwarantanny COVID-19".* Kraków: Instytut Socjologii i Filozofii UP. https://mlodziez.krakow.pl/wp-content/uploads/2020/04/Krakowska-m%C5%82odziez-COVID19.pdf

Domagała-Zyśk, E. (Ed.). (2020). *Zdalne uczenie się i nauczanie a specjalne potrzeby edukacyjne. Z doświadczeń pandemii Covid-19.* Wydawnictwo Episteme.

Doucet, A., Netolicky, D., Timmers, K., Tuscano, J. (2020). *Thinking about pedagogy in an unfolding pandemic, an independent report on approaches to distance learning during Covid-19 school closures.* https://issuu.com/educationinternational/docs/2020_research_Covid-19_eng

Dscout. (2016). *Mobile touches: Dscout's inaugural study on humans and their tech.* https://blog.dscout.com/mobile-touches [13.05.2021].

Duke, É., & Montag, C. (2017). Smartphone addiction, daily interruptions and self-reported productivity. *Addictive Behaviors Reports, 6*, 90–95. https://doi.org/10.1016/j.abrep.2017.07.002

Fundacja Szkoła z Klasą. (2021). *Rozmawiaj z Klasą. Zdrowie Psychiczne uczniów i uczennic oczami nauczycieli i nauczycielek.* Raport z badania, Warszawa: Fundacja Szkoła z Klasą.

Gajderowicz, T., & Jakubowski, M. (2020). *Cyfrowe wyzwania stojące przed polską edukacją.* Polski Instytut Ekonomiczny.

Gambin, M., Woźniak-Prus, M., Sękowski, M., & Cudo, A. (2020). Factors related to positive experiences in parent-child relationship during the COVID-19 lockdown. The role of empathy, emotions regulation, parenting self-efficacy and social support. *PsyArXiv.* https://doi.org/10.31234/osf.io/yhtqa

Gustafsson, E., Thomee, S., Grimby-Ekman, A., & Hagberg, M. (2017). Texting on mobile phones and musculoskeletal disorders in young adults: A five-year cohort study. *Applied Ergonomics, 58*, 208–214. https://doi.org/10.1016/j.apergo.2016.06.012

Harding, S., Morris, R., Gunnell, D., Ford, T., Hollingworth, W., Tilling, K., Evans, R., Bell, S., Grey, J., Brockman, R., Campbell, R., Araya, R., Murphy, S., & Kidger, J. (2019). Is teachers' mental health and well-being associated with students' mental health and well-being? *Journal of Affective Disorders, 1*(242), 180–187. https://doi.org/10.1016/j.jad.2018.08.080. Epub 2018 Aug 17.

Kułaga, A. (2020). Zdalne nauczanie uczniów z niepełnosprawnością intelektualną w stopniu umiarkowanym. In E. Domagała-Zyśk (Ed.), *Zdalne uczenie się i nauczanie a specjalne potrzeby edukacyjne. Z doświadczeń pandemii Covid-19.* Wydawnictwo Episteme.

Lanaj, K., Johnson, R. E., & Barnes, C. M. (2014). Beginning the workday yet already depleted? Consequences of late-night smartphone use and sleep. *Organizational Behavior and Human Decision Processes, 124*(1), 11–23. https://doi.org/10.1016/j.obhdp.2014.01.001

Lewandowska, P. (2020). Dostępność edukacji zdalnej dla uczniów z niepełnosprawnością słuchową w klasach IV–VIII. In E. Domagała-Zyśk (Ed.), *Zdalne uczenie się i nauczanie a specjalne potrzeby edukacyjne. Z doświadczeń pandemii Covid-19.* Wydawnictwo Episteme.

Makaruk, K., Włodarczyk, J., & Skoneczna, P. (2019). *Problematyczne używanie internetu przez młodzież.* Raport z badań. Warszawa: Fundacja Dajemy Dzieciom Siłę. https://fdds.pl/_Resources/Persistent/d/1/6/4/d164e2f03eba3e6195f1dae6da1934177afedfe0/Problematyczne-uzywanie-internetu-przez-mlodziez-Raport-z-badan.pdf [13.05.2021].

Makaruk, K., Włodarczyk, J., & Szredzińska, R. (2020). *Negatywne doświadczenia młodzieży w trakcie pandemii. Raport z badań ilościowych.* Fundacja Dajemy Dzieciom Siłę.

Murphy, M. P. A. (2020). Covid-19 and emergency eLearning: Consequences of the securitization of higher education for post-pandemic pedagogy. *Contemporary Security Policy, 41*(3), 492–505.

Oberle, E., Ji, X. R., Kerai, S., Guhn, M., Schonert-Reichl, K. A., & Gadermann, A. M. (2020). Screen time and extracurricular activities as risk and protective factors for mental health in adolescence: A population-level study. *Preventive Medicine, 141*, 106291.

Ostaszewski, K., Bobrowski, K., Borucka, A., Kocoń, K., Okulicz-Kozaryn, K., & Pisarska, A. (2005). *Raport techniczny z realizacji projektu badawczego p.n. Monitorowanie trendów używania substancji psychoaktywnych oraz wskaźników innych wybranych aspektów zdrowia psychicznego u młodzieży szkolnej.* Instytut Psychiatrii i Neurologii w Warszawie. https://www.researchgate.net/publication/270276040

Pisula, E., Pankowski, D., Nowakowska, I., Banasiak, A., Wytrychiewicz-Pankowska, K., Markiewicz, M., & Jórczak, A. (2020). *Nauczyciele w sytuacji powrotu do szkół w czasie pandemii SARS-CoV-2. Raport z badań przeprowadzonych od 10 września do 10 października 2020.* Open Science Framework. https://doi.org/10.17605/OSF.IO/6ZNCE. https://osf.io/6znce/

Plichta, P. (2020). Różne konteksty nierówności cyfrowych a wyzwania dla zdalnej edukacji – propozycje rozwiązań. In J. Pyżalski (Ed.), *Edukacja w czasach pandemii wirusa Covid-19. Z dystansem o tym, co robimy obecnie jako nauczyciele.* EduAkcja. Pobrano z zdalnie.edu-akcja.pl.

Plichta, P., Pyżalski, J., Walter, N., Lewandowska-Walter, A., & Michałek-Kwiecień, J. (2020). Obawy, wyzwania i jasne strony pandemii – analiza tematyczna wypowiedzi studentów z niepełnosprawnościami i problemami zdrowotnymi. „Niepełnosprawność i Rehabilitacja" 3.

Ptaszek, G., Stunża, G. D., Pyżalski, J., Dębski, M., & Bigaj, M. (2020). *Edukacja zdalna: co stało się z uczniami, ich rodzicami i nauczycielami?* Gdańskie Wydawnictwo Psychologiczne.

Pyżalski, J. (Ed.). (2020). *Edukacja w czasach pandemii wirusa COVID-19. Z dystansem o tym, co robimy obecnie jako nauczyciele.* EduAkcja. https://zdalnie.edu-akcja.pl/

Pyżalski, J. (2020a). Ważne relacje uczniów i nauczycieli w czasie edukacji zdalnej. In G. Ptaszek, G. D. Stunża, J. Pyżalski, M. Dębski, & M. Bigaj (Eds.), *Edukacja zdalna: co stało się z uczniami ich rodzicami i nauczycielami?* GWP.

Pyżalski, J. (2020b). Zmiany w zakresie czasu poświęconego wybranym aktywnościom w czasie pandemii. In G. Ptaszek, G. D. Stunża, J. Pyżalski, M. Dębski, & M. Bigaj (Eds.), *Edukacja zdalna: co stało się z uczniami ich rodzicami i nauczycielami?* Gdańsk.

Pyżalski, J., Merecz, D. (red.) (2010). Psychospołeczne warunki pracy polskich nauczycieli. Pomiędzy wypaleniem zawodowym a zaangażowaniem, : Oficyna Wydawnicza „Impuls".

Pyżalski, J., & Poleszak, W. (2020). Relacje przede wszystkim – nawet jeśli obecnie tylko zapośredniczone. In W. J. Pyżalski (Ed.), *Edukacja w czasach pandemii wirusa COVID-19. Z dystansem o tym, co robimy obecnie jako nauczyciele* (pp. 51–58). EduAkcja. https://zdalnie.edu-akcja.pl/

Pyżalski, J., Zdrodowska, A., Tomczyk, Ł., & Abramczuk, K. (2019). *Polskie badanie EU Kids Online 2018. Najważniejsze wyniki i wnioski.* Wydawnictwo Naukowe UAM.

Romiszowski, A., & Mason, R. (1986). Computer-mediated communication. In D. Jonassen (Ed.), *Handbook of research for educational communications and technology* (pp. 438–456). Simon and Schuster Macmillan.

Rosen, L. D., Carrier, L. M., & Cheever, N. A. (2013). Facebook and texting made me do it: Media-induced task-switching while studying. *Computers in Human Behavior, 29*(3), 948–958. https://doi.org/10.1016/j.chb.2012.12.001

Ruszkowska, M. (2020). Funkcjonowanie placówek opiekuńczo-wychowawczych w czasie pandemii. *Problemy Opiekuńczo-Wychowawcze, 595*, 67–75.

Ryan, N. D. (2005). Treatment of depression in children and adolescents. *Lancet, 366*, 933–940.

Schnauber-Stockmann, A., Meier, A., & Reinecke, L. (2018). Procrastination out of habit? The role of impulsive versus reflective media selection in procrastinatory media use. *Media Psychology, 21*(4), 640–668. https://doi.org/10.1080/15213269.2018.1476156

Sewall, C. J., Bear, T. M., Merranko, J., & Rosen, D. (2020). How psychosocial well-being and usage amount predict inaccuracies in retrospective estimates of digital technology use. *Mobile Media & Communication, 8*(3), 379–399. https://doi.org/10.1177/2050157920902830

Sikorska, I., Lipp, N., Wróbel, P., & Wyra, M. (2021). Adolescent mental health and activities in the period of social isolation caused by the Covid-19 pandemic. *Postępy Psychiatrii i Neurologii, 30,* 79–95.

Smahel, D., Machackova, H., Mascheroni, G., Dedkova, L., Staksrud, E., Ólafsson, K., Livingstone, S., & Hasebrink, U. (2020). EU kids online 2020: Survey results from 19 countries. *EU Kids Online.* https://doi.org/10.21953/lse.47fdeqj01ofo

Stunża, G. (2020). Zdania (nie)dokończone. Edukacja zdalna w wypowiedziach uczniów, rodziców i nauczycieli. Jakościowy moduł badawczy. In G. Ptaszek, G. D. Stunża, J. Pyżalski, M. Dębski, & M. Bigaj (Eds.), *Edukacja zdalna: co stało się z uczniami ich rodzicami i nauczycielami?* GWP.

Sultana, A., Tasnim, S., Hossain, M. M., Bhattacharya, S., & Purohit, N. (2021). Digital screen time during the Covid-19 pandemic: A public health concern. *F1000Research, 10*(81), 81.

United Nations. (2020). *Policy brief: Education during Covid-19 and Beyond.* https://www.un.org/development/desa/dspd/wp0content/uploads/sites/22/2020/08/sg_policy_brief_Covid-19_and_education_august_2020.pdf.99

Vanden Abeele, M. M. (2020). Digital Well-being as a dynamic construct. *Communication Theory.* https://doi.org/10.1093/ct/qtaa024

Walter, N. (2020). Mamy (za) duży wybór – jak nie zgubić się wśród narzędzi cyfrowych? In J. Pyżalski (Ed.), *Edukacja w czasach pandemii wirusa COVID-19 Z dystansem o tym, co robimy obecnie jako nauczyciele* (pp. 51–58). EduAkcja. https://zdalnie.edu-akcja.pl/

Walter, N., & Pyzalski, J. (2022). Lessons learned from Covid-19 emergency remote education. Adaptation to crisis distance education of teachers by developing new or modified digital competences. In Ł. Tomczyk & L. Fedeli (Eds.), *Digital literacy for teachers.* Springer Nature.

Jacek Pyżalski is an experienced project coordinator (over 20 national and international projects concerning education—among them 8 directly on the use of ICT by young people) and a member of national and international scientific project teams (over 60 projects). He has been also a Polish representative in three European Science Foundation Actions—COST IS0801 (cyberbullying) and IS 2010 (appearance impact), which all consider social aspects of education and health education also in terms of the new media. Prof. Pyżalski has published many articles on new media in education, including both risks and opportunities, and is interested in constructive involvement of ICT in contemporary didactics in educational practice. Some of his works are highly cited by the international research community. In 2018, he received the prestigious Tomasz Hofmokl Prize in the "Information Society" category. The award was presented during the jubilee gala organized on the occasion of the 25th anniversary of the Scientific and Academic Computer Network—State Research Institution.

Natalia Walter is a graduate of media pedagogy (media education), as well as integrated pre-school and early-school education. Head of the Department of Media Education at the Faculty of Educational Studies at Adam Mickiewicz University in Poznań, specialist in ICT and media education, social support (mainly online), and e-learning. For many years, she has worked with people with disabilities, which is why she also researches how the media can support people in a difficult life situation. For several years, she has worked with children and teens as an IT teacher and currently conducts media education workshops for students, teachers, and parents. Dean's Representative for e-Learning at the Faculty of Educational Studies, member of the Adam Mickiewicz University Distance Learning Council. Author of books and articles on new media, ICT education, e-learning, and online social support.

Chapter 8
Impact of the Covid-19 Pandemic on the Well-being of Children with Disabilities and their Parents in Azerbaijan

Tunzala Verdiyeva, Aygun Muradli, and Nargiz Huseynova

Abstract Although the Coronavirus Epidemic, which affects the world today, affects every individual in the society, those who are most exposed to the negative conditions of the epidemic are children with disabilities and their families. There are many reasons why people in this group are more affected by the epidemic than others. Families with children, especially those with disabled children face a lot of stress due to the interruption of psychological and economic support. During the Covid-19 pandemic, children with disabilities and their parents experienced increased symptoms of stress.

The impact of social isolation or social exclusion on children's well-being, including concerns about increased anxiety, depression, stress, and exacerbation or recurrence of pre-existing mental health problems, is widespread. Quarantine restrictions and the overall burden on families, as well as children with disabilities, can lead to discrimination.

Newly collected data on the effects of Covid-19 should contribute to the redesign of data collection methodologies to address the challenges faced by children with disabilities. The measures taken to protect Azerbaijan from the pandemic have made for a challenging process. Different methods to deal with the sanitary crisis in the region have resulted in different negative impacts such as the fight against pandemic and the effect it has had on the psychology of people and the psychological impact of prevention measures on people. Disabled children and their parents have been one of the most impacted groups during the pandemic. The impact of the pandemic on this vulnerable group primarily means difficulties in their socialization and social integration. Unusual social communication and self-service skills have disappeared as day care centres and community-based rehabilitation centres ceased their activities visually and moved online with inclusive education classes.

T. Verdiyeva (✉) · A. Muradli · N. Huseynova
Azerbaijan University, Baku, Azerbaijan
e-mail: tunzala.verdiyeva@au.edu.az

© The Author(s), under exclusive license to Springer Nature Switzerland AG 2022
L. Dalingwater et al. (eds.), *The Unequal Costs of Covid-19 on Well-being in Europe*,
Human Well-Being Research and Policy Making,
https://doi.org/10.1007/978-3-031-14425-7_8

133

The chapter examines the impact of the Covid-19 pandemic on vulnerable groups in the world and more specifically in Azerbaijan, as well as on the health, psycho-social status, and socialization of children with disabilities. The chapter studies the activities of international organizations such as the UN, UNICEF, UAFA working with the children with disabilities and also local organizations such as Joint and Healthy Public Union during the Covid-19 pandemic, and evaluates their activities through interviews with the heads of these organizations. The opinions of parents of children with special needs were also taken into consideration and the problems faced by children and families were analysed.

8.1 Background

Azerbaijan is a state which became independent after the collapse of the Soviet system. The Soviet history has left a legacy in the mind of the people and also in the management systems. In some cases, one can observe tensions in the social support system and its organization which is generated by the past. The Republic of Azerbaijan is a transcontinental country located on the border of Eastern Europe and Western Asia. It is part of the South Caucasus region and is bordered by the Caspian Sea to the east, Russia (Republic of Dagestan) to the north, Georgia to the northwest, Armenia and Turkey to the west, and Iran to the south.

On 18 October 1991, Azerbaijan regained its independence and as a newly independent nation, Azerbaijan continued to develop in many areas of life. The newly independent country interacted with a number of government agencies around the world. An example of this is the socio-economic measures taken by government agencies to reduce the impact of the Covid-19 pandemic during the study. Azerbaijan is a member of the UN, Council of Europe, Organization for Security and Cooperation in Europe, GUAM, Eastern Partnership, Turkic Council, Organization of Islamic Cooperation, International Monetary Fund, Asian Development Bank, European Bank for Reconstruction and Development, Black Sea Economic Cooperation Organization, IAEA, and Chemical Weapons Prohibition. It is a member of the Organization of NATO's Partnership for Peace (PfP).

8.2 Context

The outbreak of the new coronavirus (Covid-19) in December 2019 started in China and it was declared a pandemic in March 2020, by the World Health Organization. It affected more than 200 countries around the world with a total number of Covid-19 patients being more than two million. A pandemic that has an unprecedented impact on almost every country in the world could lead to catastrophic social, economic, and political crises. People lost their jobs and their income at a time when it is impossible to predict when normal life will return. The Covid-19 pandemic has also affected disabled children and their families socio-economically and psychologically (Yousaf et al., 2020).

The effects on Azerbaijan were more than 792,216 patients contaminated and 9703 deaths till 10 April 2022 (https://koronavirusinfo.az/az/page/statistika/azerbaycanda-cari-veziyyet).

8.3   The Situation of Children with Disabilities During the Covid-19 Pandemic

The Covid-19 pandemic has had significant psychological and health impacts on the global population (Yousaf et al., 2020). The increased stress and anxiety associated with acquiring the life-threatening disease was further compounded by the loneliness and enforced social isolation of quarantine, particularly in children and adolescents. Research from past pandemics has found that these disease-containment responses can be traumatizing to a significant proportion of children and parents (Dalton et al., 2020). Although the number of children affected by the disease is small, and most of the affected children show only mild symptoms, the disease and the containment measures are likely to negatively impact on the mental health and well-being of children. Even though children all over the world are likely to be affected, those with disabilities, living in slums, isolation centres, and conflicts zones are likely to be at a greater risk (Yousaf et al., 2020).

The responses of a child to a crisis situation depend upon his prior exposure to emergency situations, his/her physical and mental health, socio-economic circumstances of the family, and cultural background (Dalton et al., 2020). Different studies have shown that crisis events negatively impact the psychological well-being of children. Anxiety, depression, disturbances in sleep, and appetite as well as impairment in social interactions are the most common presentations. A recent study conducted in China screened children and adolescents for behavioural and emotional distress due to the Covid-19 pandemic. Clinginess, distraction, irritability, and fear that family members can contract the deadly disease were the most common behavioural problems identified (Jiao et al., 2020). The Covid-19 pandemic has significant psychological and health effects on the global population (Brooks et al., 2020).

Children with disabilities are even more vulnerable, not just because of their underlying health conditions but because of the social circumstances in which they live. They are more likely to be poor, more commonly of minority race (and as such experience the negative impacts of structural and personally mediated racism more frequently than their non-disabled peers), and some have a higher risk of contracting Covid-19 (Bandi et al., 2020). Also, they and their families routinely face stigma and discrimination, often with multiple intersecting identities that are associated with exacerbated inequalities (Green et al., 2005).

Children with disabilities and their families are dealing with the loss of home nursing, therapies, educational supports, personal protective equipment, other medical supplies, informal caregiving from extended family members, and safe access to medical providers. Delayed or forgone care during the pandemic is a source of concern in pediatrics (Collins et al., 2020) and likely disproportionately impacts children with disabilities who historically have had more health care concerns and unmet needs. The closure of schools, childcare centres, and other community organizations has limited community partners' abilities to detect and report abuse/neglect (Campbell, 2020). Additional vulnerabilities exist for children with disabilities living in skilled nursing or other congregate care facilities due to the high rate of transmission in these types of settings (Collins et al., 2020). Families who have children residing in institutional settings have been worried about the risk of Covid-19 spreading through facilities and the loss of visitations, thus they are faced with the challenging decision to abruptly try to integrate their children with extensive needs into their homes without appropriate support to ensure well-being (Goldman et al., 2020).

Children with neurodevelopmental problems such as attention deficit/hyperactivity disorder (ADHD), autism spectrum disorder (ASD), cognitive impairment, Tourette syndrome and children with developmental disabilities or NDD may be particularly vulnerable to stress due to significant changes in routine and service access. Changes include reducing the availability of official and informal support, including inability to attend school and limited contact with immediate or long-term family members (Sprang & Silman, 2013).

Changes in service delivery, including health care, during a pandemic may pose additional challenges in addressing the routine health needs of children which is expected to be exaggerated in children with NDDs. As health services close down non-critical aspects of delivery, children are likely to miss out on access to standard care such as routine health checks. Families may also be reluctant to attend health facilities for fear of exposure to Covid-19 or due to reluctance to be a burden on already-stretched health services. This may bring unintended consequences such as families increasing child medication dosage without medical input or monitoring. Substantial reductions in the availability of therapeutic supports conventionally delivered through face-to-face sessions (e.g. behavioural interventions) are also likely to adversely impact children with NDDs and their parents (Thornton, 2020).

Families may also be reluctant to go to health institutions for fear of Covid-19 exposure or unwilling to burden an already deficient level of healthcare. This can have unintended consequences, for example, if families increase the child drug dose without medical input or monitoring.

8.4   Parental Stress

Many families are isolated at home, under great stress, and unable to receive in-person support. Confinement, social isolation, and inability to use familiar coping mechanisms like taking personal space, visiting with family/friends, or going to mall or movie theatre, dining out, or going for a long drive on car or motorcycle with spouse or friend may exacerbate the impact of these stressors.

Stable, supportive, and nurturing caregiver relationship offers young children fostering trust, positive social-emotional development, and the capacity to form a secure and strong relationship in the future (Honig, 2002). Extensive research shows that fear can be contagious and children are extremely sensitive to the emotional state of the adults around them, who are their essential source of security and emotional well-being. The pandemic has disrupted the financial and economic activities around the world creating a sense of uncertainty among the masses. A survey conducted in the USA indicates high level of psychological distress among people suffering from financial losses. Around 40% of the people with children less than 12 years of age fall into high distress group and are having difficulties in dealing with their work responsibilities and childcare. More than 50% of the parents have reported that financial troubles due to social isolation are affecting their parenting skills (Imran et al., 2020).

8.5   Disabled Children in Azerbaijan Faced with Covid-19

In order to reduce the impact of the Covid-19 pandemic on children with disabilities and their families in Azerbaijan, a number of activities have been carried out in government, non-governmental organizations and local private organizations. One of these measures and decisions is the decision made by the Prime Minister of the Republic of Azerbaijan during the Covid-19 pandemic.

8.6   Decision of the Cabinet of Ministers of the Republic of Azerbaijan

On prolongation of disability of persons with disabilities in the fight against a new type of coronavirus (Covid-19) pandemic

Guided by the eighth paragraph of Article 119 of the Constitution of the Republic of Azerbaijan, to ensure social protection of persons with disabilities in the fight against a new type of coronavirus (Covid-19) pandemic the Cabinet of Ministers of the Republic of Azerbaijan resolves:

1. The period of disability of persons with disabilities, including children with disabilities under 18 years of age, whose period of disability expires on March 1, 2020, is limited to

the period of special quarantine in the territory of the Republic of Azerbaijan until July 1, 2020. in the regions (cities) where hardening is applied, it should be extended until the end of the hardening period.
2. To the Ministry of Labor and Social Protection of the population of the Azerbaijan Republic to solve the questions following from this Resolution.

Ali Asadov
Prime Minister of the Republic of Azerbaijan
Baku city, April, 7, 2020
No.128 [23].
https://e-qanun.az/framework/44866

During the Covid-19 pandemic, a number of organizations worked with children with special needs and their families. One of these was the State Committee on Family, Women and Children. Organized by the State Committee on Family, Women and Children, measures were taken to protect children's rights, introduce talented children to the society, work with children, effectively use their free time, and implement measures related to Covid-19 and special quarantine rules. Important work has been done to ensure compliance with the rules of the regime and awareness-raising activities have been carried out.

Protecting children from the violence they may face in society, and empowering them to know and protect their rights is one of the most pressing issues today. For this purpose, on 9 January 2021, the Committee held an event with the participation of children. The children spoke about their rights and issues of concern and made suggestions. Emphasizing the important role of parents and adults in the safety of children, the importance of being more active in protecting the rights of children was noted.

In particular, the implementation of awareness-raising and control measures to protect children from violence in the regions, the activities with families to respect the views of children, mass propaganda campaigns to instil respect for every child in society, tightening legislation to punish crimes against children put forward proposals.

During the Covid-19 pandemic, people refrained from donating blood and going to hospitals, and a number of government agencies and associations called on people to donate blood to people suffering from blood diseases. In response to the Heydar Aliyev Foundation's call, a blood donation campaign was held at the National Hematology and Transphysiology Center on 7 April 2021 at the initiative of the State Committee for Family, Women and Children's Affairs to support registered children in need of monthly blood transfusions and increase their blood supply. Employees of "Hopeful Future" Youth Organization, "Birlik" Charitable Organization, "Azerbaijan Women's Republican Society" Public Union, "SAF For the Sake of Life" Youth Public Union, Baku Textile Factory, Azerbaijan Women's Entrepreneurship Development Association, Azerbaijan-Turkey Businessmen's Union took part in the humanist action. And members, volunteer families also attended. At the call of the committee, 399 people joined the action.

On 29 April 2021, the Committee held a live online discussion for parents on "Psychological rehabilitation of children with disabilities during restrictions".

During the online meeting, the psychologist of the Committee, the Center for Public Health and Reforms, as well as the Rehabilitation Center for People with Down Syndrome answered questions from parents about the rehabilitation and social adaptation of children with disabilities.

8.7 Activities of Child and Family Support Centres

In 2020, during the Covid-19 pandemic, 11 Child and Family Support Centres under the State Committee for Family, Women and Children's Affairs continued to operate in accordance with the rules of quarantine and social isolation. During the current year, the centres working to identify at-risk families, assessing their socio-psychological situation, a comprehensive approach to solving family problems, resolving complaints received directly or jointly by relevant agencies, domestic violence, violence against women and children, early work has been done on marriages, girls' school dropouts, public awareness campaigns to promote human rights in general, and other important areas.

As part of the "Family to Family" campaign organized by the Committee, 146 families provided assistance to 745 vulnerable families. The State Customs Committee and the "Easy Volunteers" organization provided food assistance to 74 elderly and lonely people, 340 people together with the Women's Resource Centers, and 145 families by the UADM. With the financial support of the European Union and UNICEF, food assistance was provided to 483 low-income and at-risk families living in communities where regional centres operate, along with UADM staff and Easy Volunteers.

The work of the committee during the Covid-19 pandemic, as well as its work with local and international organizations, is commendable.

8.8 Analysis of the Impact of the Covid-19 Pandemic on Families

The State Committee for Family, Women and Children's Affairs conducted an analysis of the situation in interpersonal relationships in families as a result of social isolation measures and the application of a special quarantine regime in the country in connection with the Covid-19 pandemic. The results of the survey once again showed that every event that took place in the environment and society negatively affected the family in one way or another.

In April 2022, in order to support the creative potential of children with autism during the April 2022 Covid-19 pandemic, the Agency for Sustainable and Opera-tional Social Security (DOST) held the event "Embrace Difference"! at the Inclusive Development and Creativity Centre. Speaking at the event, Minister of Labor and

Social Protection Sahil Babayev spoke about the attention and care for this category of people in Azerbaijan, emphasizing the importance of such events in the integration of children with autism into society.

During the event, participants witnessed one child Hussein's ability to lead, despite his autism. They enjoyed the memorable concert programme of the newly created inclusive chamber orchestra at the centre, the classical music presented, especially the music played by the visually impaired Farid Abdullayev on the national instrument tar.

At the meetings of the Agency for Sustainable and Operational Social Security (DOST) in 2020, information was provided on the work done by the state in the field of protection of the rights of persons with disabilities, including the goals and objectives of the state. In the meetings held regarding the action plan for 2020 and its implementation, the proposed methodology of tracking and monitoring methods during the pandemic was put out for public discussion for the study of opinions and suggestions.

8.9 Report of the Ministry of Labour and Social Protection of the Population of the Azerbaijan Republic for 2020

Continuation of assistance to the families (individuals) whom the State targeted social assistance (TSA) was disbanded, although the special restriction regime was extended till the end of the special quarantine regime and simplification of the appointment of TSS during this period covered 38.9 thousand members of 9.4 thousand families and local currency 8.6 mln. manats were spent. In addition to the above, from March 1, 2020, the period of disability of persons with disabilities, including children under 18 years of age, whose term of disability expires, has been extended due to the special quarantine regime in the territory of the Republic of Azerbaijan.

8.10 Social Services Agency

In 2021, a total of 2200 people were provided with social services in social service institutions subordinated to the Agency for Social Services. It served 368 children with disabilities in social service institutions, 245 elderly people in social service institutions, 538 people in psychoneurological social service institutions, shelters for vulnerable groups and 332 people in social rehabilitation institutions.

A number of organizations including the United Nations International Children's Emergency Fund (UNICEF) and United Aid for Azerbaijan (UAFA) have been active in Azerbaijan in developing strong communicative network to disseminate the consequences of the Covid-19 pandemic through conferences and other public comments. For instance, UNICEF Azerbaijan urged parents and a number of institutions to address the nature of the pandemic and take significant steps: UNICEF argued that comprehensive measures are required to protect children's safety, well-being, and the future from Covid-19 [21]. In particular, it has raised a number of important issues for children, which go beyond the direct threats posed by Covid-19 and according to UNICEF Representative in Azerbaijan Edward Carwardine, most of these issues are already being dealt with by close cooperation between UNICEF and the government.

> We know that children and families will feel the impact of Covid-19 in many areas of their lives—Daily Health and Nutrition, General and Early Education, Protecting Children from Family Violence and Long-Term Isolation Focusing on Psychological Tension as well as economic impact on vulnerable groups in communities—in Azerbaijan, UNICEF is already working with government and civil society partners to minimize the risks in all these areas, he said.

Children with disabilities and their families, as well as people without disabilities, benefited from UNICEF-supported efforts during the Covid-19 pandemic. Simple preventive measures, especially hand-washing guides, have reached more than one million people in the country through video and direct communication with people with Internet access. "Regional Development" Public Union - Azerbaijan (RDPU) prepared the materials and supported their online and physical distribution, and during this period the support of UNICEF was carried out with the help of the government of Azerbaijan. UNICEF has even offered cooperation through the Government of Azerbaijan to disseminate practical information about children and their nutrition and online advice to parents on children's health, nutrition and early development. In the case just mentioned to the Ministry of Health's Public Health and Reforms Center, the State Compulsory Health Insurance Institution and the Ministry of Health were all involved. UNICEF also supports the Ministry of Labor and Social Protection to investigate the socio-economic impact of the virus on vulnerable families, with particular support for single parents, families whose children have been returned from government institutions. In addition, UNICEF, in partnership with the Ministry and ASAN Service Volunteers, initially offered to support the provision of food packages to 1000 particularly vulnerable families.

8.11 An Investigation into Agency of Two Azerbaijani organizations in Support of Children

The remainder of this paper examines how Azerbaijan's aid agencies support the challenges faced by children. The views of leading members of key support agencies are presented through interviews.

8.11.1 Autism Center of the Together and Healthy Public Union

We first considered children with autism spectrum disorders.

The head of "Autism Center of the Together and Healthy Public Union", Ayten Eynalova, was interviewed on 31 January 2022 and spoke about the impact of the Covid-19 pandemic on children with autism spectrum disorders and their parents. She explained that the "Autism Center" was established with the support of the Heydar Aliyev foundation and has been operating since 2013 after state registration. Since that year, the main goal of the Center has been to support people diagnosed with autism spectrum disorders and their families, as well as to implement awareness-raising projects in the field of autism in the country.

The Autism Center currently has a rehabilitation centre. There are about 90 people with autism spectrum disorders in this rehabilitation centre between the ages of 0 and 25. There is also a cafe and workshop called "Kashalata". The purpose of the Kashalata cafe is to attract teenagers and young people with autism to vocational training and employment. Employees of Kashalata cafe and workshop are also teenagers and young people with autism. The main goal here is to involve children with autism spectrum disorders in this process as they get older.

Eynalova emphasizes that they currently work with about 40 specialists who intervene in the development of children through a science-based system called ABBA (Applied Behavior Analysis). At this centre, a specialist works with each child with autism spectrum disorder, and in this individual process, all the graphical, data records are taken and fixed for the recording and results of this system. She adds that they attract students and specialists to the centre. They can practice at the centre as it presents affordable conditions for the higher qualified specialists in Azerbaijan.

Eynalova continued that, as part of the BP project, they are implementing career planning for about 40 teenagers and young people with autism spectrum disorders. And as a result of this career planning, they provide them with vocational training support, and by meeting with companies, they plan to involve each individual with at least 10 autism spectrum disorders based on this project by extracting an individual education plan for each child. In addition, they have created a web portal autizmportali.az (https://www.autizmportali.az/). Through this portal, they have posted about 100 scientifically based methodical videos, videos of the teaching process, and educational videos. Anyone who is an Internet user not only in the capital Baku, but also in many other regions can support their children by watching those videos, and they have also posted many educational topics. They have written more than one million books, adapted books to the country, and created resources in our native language. And in this regard, they have uploaded the pdf format of our books, which they have written and translated, to this web portal so that it is accessible to everyone and everyone can use them. Conferences, seminars, and social activities, which are fashion shows, marches performed by our children, awareness-raising campaigns in shopping malls, etc., work are being done.

This was why Eynalova explained that the centre's staff only stayed at home for a month and a half while working online in all businesses in the country. Then they appealed to the government and said that home closure has a negative impact on the development of children with autism spectrum disorders, and they continued the work process after the permit, because they have a special process, the work process is not in a group format, so people with special needs, such as children stay at home. As a result of the application, with the permission of the state, they resumed their work after a maximum of one and a half months of strict quarantine.

"Autism Center of the Together and Healthy Public Union" held more than 20 seminars during that month and a half. These were particularly important for family just starting out and where the family was unable to intervene in the home process and solve the problems they were facing. They taught them how to deal with this process through these workshops. The center also holds educational sessions for individuals with high-functioning autism who continue their learning online. For such student, the results were obvious as long as the learning process followed the methodology developed for such purposes However, of course, this does not apply to all people with autism spectrum disorders. A child with a severe autism spectrum disorder needs face-to-face and individual training, but online contact did prevent them from becoming aggressive.

Eynalova said that the number of children suffering from the Covid-19 pandemic did not exceed 10. She concluded that the whole world was experiencing the same thing and they had to learn over time how to deal with it and how to approach this new situation. The centre has learned that overcoming the pandemic was possible by actually socializing children more individually not by shutting them down. The greatest difficulty for people with autism is maintaining social distance, because children with autism are not very sociable people, and when you try and compel such children to do something, you face an additional problem. We have been keeping that distance for years, we have been keeping it from birth for many years, but we knew that new socializations were needed here. At the same time, they are already teaching them how to spend more functional time with their children if such a situation occurs again.

In closing the interview Eynalova said "we advise parents to get a result from each situation. Let's organize more seminars for them, give them advice on reading books, support them to develop themselves".

8.11.2   United Aid For Azerbaijan (UAFA)

UAFA staff member, doctor, child development specialist, CHED (Child Health, Education, Social Development) and teacher Ulviya Mirzayeva spoke about United Aid For Azerbaijan (UAFA) assistance to Azerbaijan in the Covid-19 pandemic for children with disabilities and their parents.

Mirzayeva said:

One of UAFA's most important missions is to promote optimism and trust through action, believing that only optimistic thinking, action and words can change everything in a complex environment. This is the main principle underlying our work and distinguishing UAFA; this optimism grows and brings us more local support, which in turn allows our organization to help more children and families.

According to Mirzayeva, UAFA also carries out activities in several areas. Of these, we have "community with rehabilitation", "community-based rehabilitation centers". Projects are being implemented in some regions, including Baku. We have community-based rehabilitation centres and early intervention centres in several regions where specialists work with children with disabilities.

At the same time, another direction is the involvement of children with disabilities in pre-school education and inclusive education. Community-based rehabilitation centres are available in 13 districts. It deals with all types of disabilities, and staff working with children with disabilities are child development specialists.

Different screening methods are used in the process of determining disability. In Azerbaijan, which is used in UAFA centres, the method called "Inter" is currently used. This is called Development Assessment and Monitoring. It is a screening method developed by Ankara University of Turkey. At the same time, the "Autism Center of the Together and Healthy Public Union" uses other examination methods and screening methods, such as Portek and Denver.

Mirzayeva emphasizes that during the acute period of the pandemic, they tried to continue their work online, even though the centres were closed. They tried to carry out this process together with parents. They continued classes through online platforms, and parents joined the process at home. The specialist instructed on this side of the screen, and the parent began to work with the child on the other side. As part of the pandemic, they also had a project called "Positive Parenting". The project "Positive Parenting" was a project related to the campaign to instil parenting skills, elements of positive parenting, how to be a positive parent, to inform parents about child development. More than 400 parents have joined this online project. At the same time, work on early intervention continued. If they compare the current period with the period of strict quarantine, then parents were afraid to bring their children to the centre because they were afraid that the children would be infected, but there were also parents who brought their children to institutions. At present, this process is back to normal.

UAFA gave recommendations on how parents can work with children at home during a pandemic, how to raise their children, that is, the centre received recommendations in this regard. UNICEF sent them reminders of precautions to take during the pandemic, and they tried to share them with parents at the centres as well. They shared on social networks to suggest how parents can work with children. It is very difficult to lock children with all types of disabilities at home during a pandemic. The centre found that it was very difficult to work with children with autism spectrum disorders and hyperactive children.

The period of the pandemic has left its mark in all areas. One of the areas hit the most was rehabilitation. In some regions, centres have even closed and the number of places where parents can apply has decreased. Socialization is very important for these children. When the centres are open, parents of children with disabilities who come there are in contact with each other and exchange ideas, which affects their communication and psychological well-being.

Mirzayeva spoke about how parents spend time with their children during the pandemic. The positive side of the pandemic was that the parents also had to work at home with their children. It was as if he began to exercise his expert skills. The process would have been more effective if the parent had some professional skills. It would have been more successful for parents to be part of the process so that they do not lag behind.

At the end of the interview, Mirzayeva added the study found that the Covid-19 pandemic affects children with disabilities and their families for a variety of reasons. We hope that the ongoing work in our country to eliminate the damage of the Covid-19 pandemic will also contribute to children with disabilities and their families.

The pandemic had a negative impact. Mirzayeva commented that:

> the children stayed at home for a long time, and our families in the regions suffered the most. Meetings with families in the regions continued only on online platforms, and this gave an opportunity to realize some of our projects. However, on the plus side, parents and children in the regions spent more time in nature and were able to involve their children with disabilities in daily activities.

The fact that the children stayed at home had a negative effect on their socialization. This has had a greater impact on children with severe mental disabilities. They also tried to organize various events for them, tried to provide video training in various formats for families who did not have access to any online platform.

During the pandemic, UAFA tried to hold meetings with parents through online platforms to continue working and checked some of the benefits of online classes. They noticed an increase in the number of children attending online art classes. The association did their best to ensure that children with disabilities were involved in all activities.

Although the Covid-19 pandemic affected both institutions, the organization tried to continue its work during this time, and its staff continued to reduce the impact of the pandemic on children's development, as we can see in the interviews above. It is hoped that the mitigation of the pandemic will lead to the re-socialization of children with disabilities.

8.12   Conclusion

Children with disabilities are disproportionately impacted by Covid-19 and the containment response. Thus, their caregivers must now adapt to increased stressors such as lack of access to needed therapies, medical supplies, and nursing care. Prior to Covid-19 these families were already marginalized, and this has only worsened during the pandemic. During the ongoing pandemic and beyond, strategies have had to be developed to ensure the health of those living in group homes, nursing facilities, other congregate care arrangements, and those children who are suddenly transitioning into their family homes. When containment strategies require physical distancing and limiting contact with individuals outside of one's immediate family, plans need to be made to ensure that families who are self-isolating are not cut off from the support and services their children need for optimal health. Development of such strategies must be done in a way that is transparent and allows for accountability and focuses on equity. The pandemic has shown the fault lines in health care delivery including the pervasive nature of inequities and racial disparities. With our heightened awareness to the problems faced by children with disabilities, their families, and their communities, paediatric rehabilitation providers and others can help advocate for system-level improvements and develop clinical strategies to assure children with disabilities get the care they need and deserve.

Thus, studying the impact of the Covid-19 pandemic on vulnerable groups in the world and in Azerbaijan, we came to the conclusion that the steps taken are not measures to reduce the negative impact on vulnerable groups. There is a need to further strengthen and coordinate the activities of local, regional, and international organizations working in this area. For this activity to be sustainable, the state needs to implement large-scale projects. It is necessary to create conditions for available services to be available to the entire population of the country.

References

Bandi, S., Nevid, M. Z., & Mahdavinia, M. (2020). African American children are at higher risk for COVID-19 infection. *Pediatric Allergy and Immunology, 31*(7), 861–864.

Brooks, S. K., Webster, R. K., Smith, L. E., Woodland, L., Wessely, S., Greenberg, N., & Rubin, G. J. (2020). The psychological impact of quarantine and how to reduce it: Rapid review of the evidence. *The Lancet, 395*(10227), 912–920.

Campbell, A. M. (2020). An increasing risk of family violence during the Covid-19 pandemic: Strengthening community collaborations to save lives. *Forensic Science International: Reports, 2*, 100089.

Collins, E. M., Tam, P. Y. I., Trehan, I., Cartledge, P., Bose, A., Lanaspa, M., et al. (2020). Strengthening health systems and improving the capacity of pediatric care centers to respond to epidemics, such as Covid-19 in resource-limited settings. *Journal of Tropical Pediatrics, 66*(4), 357–365.

Dalton, L., Rapa, E., & Stein, A. (2020). Protecting the psychological health of children through effective communication about Covid-19. *The Lancet Child & Adolescent Health, 4*(5), 346–347.

Green, S., Davis, C., Karshmer, E., Marsh, P., & Straight, B. (2005). Living stigma: The impact of labeling, stereotyping, separation, status loss, and discrimination in the lives of individuals with disabilities and their families. *Sociological Inquiry, 75*(2), 197–215.

Goldman, P. S., van Ijzendoorn, M. H., Sonuga-Barke, E. J., Bakermans-Kranenburg, M. J., Bradford, B., Christopoulos, A., et al. (2020). The implications of COVID-19 for the care of children living in residential institutions. *The Lancet Child & Adolescent Health, 4*(6), e12.

Honig, A. S. (2002). *Secure relationships: Nurturing infant/toddler attachment in early care settings*. National Association for the Education of Young Children, 1509 16th Street, NW, Washington, DC 20036-1426 (NAEYC order no. 123, $8).

Imran, N., Zeshan, M., & Pervaiz, Z. (2020). Mental health considerations for children & adolescents in Covid-19 pandemic. *Pakistan Journal of Medical Sciences, 36*, S67.

Jiao, W. Y., Wang, L. N., Liu, J., Fang, S. F., Jiao, F. Y., Pettoello-Mantovani, M., & Somekh, E. (2020). Behavioral and emotional disorders in children during the Covid-19 epidemic. *The Journal of Pediatrics, 221*, 264–266.

Sprang, G., & Silman, M. (2013). Posttraumatic stress disorder in parents and youth after health-related disasters. *Disaster Medicine and Public Health Preparedness, 7*(1), 105–110.

Thornton, J. (2020). Covid-19: Millions of women and children at risk as visits to essential services plummet. *BMJ, 369*, m2171.

Yousaf, M., Zahir, S., Riaz, M., Hussain, S. M., & Shah, K. (2020). Statistical analysis of forecasting Covid-19 for upcoming month in Pakistan. *Chaos, Solitons & Fractals, 138*, 109926.

https://www.unicef.org/azerbaijan/az/press-relizl%C9%99r/unicef-Covid-19-pandemiyas%C4%B1ndan-u%C5%9Faqlar%C4%B1n-t%C9%99hl%C3%BCk%C9%99sizliyini-rifah%C4%B1n%C4%B1-v%C9%99-g%C9%99l%C9%99c%C9%99yini

http://uafa.az/uafa/

https://e-qanun.az/framework/44866

http://scfwca.gov.az/store/media/Aila%20qadin%20ushaq%20Jurnal%C4%B1.pdf

http://dost.gov.az/news/388

http://dost.gov.az/news/203

https://sosial.gov.az/uploads/files/2022/03/illik-hesabat-2020.pdf

https://sosial.gov.az/uploads/files/2022/03/illik-hesabat-2021.pdf

Tunzala Verdiyeva has a Doctor of Philosophy in Pedagogy. She worked as a psychologist at high schools in Baku from 2001 to 2016. She was a lecturer on a Social Work Refresher Program at Baku Institute of Retraining of Pedagogical Personnel (2010–2012) and a lecturer in Psychology at the Baku Institute of Retraining of Pedagogical Personnel (2010–2014) at Baku State University. She also lectured in the Sociology Department at Azerbaijan University (2012–2014) and the Organization of Social Work Department (2014–2017). She was appointed a senior lecturer in 2017 in the Organization of Social Work Department, Azerbaijan University. Since 2019, she is a head of the Organization of Social Work Department. She was awarded the "Tereqqi" Award (No. 1-693) by President Ilham Aliyev's decree No 1133 of October 4 in 2010 and has obtained several research grants including the Organization of Events on Promoting Patriotism in Secondary Schools in Baku Project by Council for State Support to Non-Governmental Organizations under the President of the Republic of Azerbaijan, Project Manager—2016.

Aygun Muradli graduated from Azerbaijan University in 2021 with a master's degree in social work. She works as a lecturer of social work at the Organization of Social Work Department.

Nargiz Huseynova has a Bachelor degree in English Language Teaching and is studying towards a Master's degree. Since 2020, she has also been working as an assistant at the Department of Foreign Languages, Azerbaijan University.

Part III
Health Inequalities and the Pandemic

Chapter 9
Lessons Learned by Health Professionals and Good Practices in Relation with Population Well-being Across Europe

Manuel Lillo-Crespo

Abstract The Covid-19 pandemic has had a huge impact on populations' health and well-being across the world since the beginning of 2020 to date. The pivot of this pandemic is a crucial element that has become almost as important as the virus itself, namely, the lockdown and its consequences such as the ones affecting population well-being understood in terms of health outcomes. Although the rationale for lockdown is grounded with strong epidemiological arguments, exploring the barely unseen consequences of the Covid-19 pandemic from the perspective of health is mandatory for the consensus of a European robust agreed position against the numerous problems associated with the SARS-CoV-2 virus as well as preventing and early-detecting future potentially similar situations. Based on the situation lived across Europe, in this chapter, we explore those consequences of the Covid-19 pandemic on population well-being studies from a health outcomes perspective. The data comprises the still unknown evidence for the scientific field that has emerged from the professional experience as the virus has spread faster than the production of scientific evidence. The aim is to give voice to the health professionals' experiences and the organizations' initiatives in Europe through the lessons they have learned in their day-to-day practice, in many cases shared with other colleagues worldwide, sometimes supported by literature published regarding this topic and organizations' strategical positions with the objective to extract those good practices on the basis of their experiential learning. A qualitative methodology approach based on a Delphi Technique was conducted with health professionals from different European regions and allied countries considered as experts who lived the different pandemic waves towards highlighting the most prevalent health problems observed. The chapter also stresses the health outcomes mainly affected according to their lived experience and the good practices, strategies and initiatives applied in their own professional settings to overcome the unknown and unexpected Covid-19 pandemic and improve positively the population well-being and health.

M. Lillo-Crespo (✉)
University of Alicante, Alicante, Spain
e-mail: manuel.lillo@ua.es

9.1 The Meaning of "Being Well", "Well-being", and "Welfare"

Well-being has been defined by different authors as the combination of feeling good and functioning well, the experience of positive emotions such as happiness and contentment as well as the development of one's potential, having some control over one's life, having a sense of purpose, and experiencing positive relationships (Huppert et al., 2009). Research into well-being and what it means to be "well" has been organized into two mainstreams of enquiry: "hedonic" well-being, which is associated with positive affect and is achieved through the pursuit of pleasure, enjoyment, and comfort, and "eudaimonic" well-being, associated with realizing ones potential and is achieved through seeking to develop the best in oneself (Huta & Ryan, 2010). Keyes et al. (2002) extend these distinctions to encompass two different traditions of research, one focused on subjective well-being which includes the evaluation of life between the balance of positive and negative affect and overall satisfaction with life (hedonic happiness), and another focused on psychological well-being which encompasses perceived thriving with regard to the existential challenges of life (eudaimonic happiness). There are researchers who dispute the need for distinct constructions of hedonic and eudaimonic happiness (Kashdan et al., 2008) and a lack of consensus in the field as to a specific definition of well-being has made research into well-being difficult to contrast and compare (Hefferon & Boniwell, 2011). However, Keyes et al. (2002) used factor analysis of data from over 3000 respondents to demonstrate that subjective well-being and psychological well-being are conceptually similar but empirically distinct. Although both concepts are applied to measuring well-being, they have different definitions of what it means to be well and so, he argues, cannot be used interchangeably (Keyes et al., 2002).

In the philosophical, psychological, and related literature on personal happiness and subjective well-being, it is common to differentiate theories of it in light of the degree to which it is thought to be a function of positive mental states. According to some theories, well-being is solely a positive state of mind, typically a matter of feeling pleasure and judging one's life to be satisfactory. In contrast, other theories maintain that well-being is not merely mental and is constituted, for instance, by conditions such as exhibiting good character, having a family, or making important achievements. The notion of subjective well-being is currently the dominant conception of happiness in psychological literature. It is currently considered to be a multidimensional construct, referring to distinct but related aspects that are often treated as a single property called happiness. Specifically, subjective well-being these days tends to encompass how people evaluate their own lives in terms of both affective, how we feel and emote, and cognitive components of well-being (Diener et al., 1999; Veenhoven, 1994) referring to what we think. Overall, high subjective well-being is seen to combine frequent and intense positive affective states, the relative absence of negative emotions, and satisfaction with one's life as a whole. It can be seen as a positive psychological experience of one's state of existence and development that is not a mere emotional flash, but is instead a stable, hedonic mood arising from conscious or unconscious judgment. The feeling or affective side of experience is a pleasant state of mind, perhaps one of enjoyment, whereas the judging or cognitive side is a matter of deeming one's life to have achieved a certain standard.

Another term used when talking about well-being is welfare. In the broadest sense, welfare refers to the well-being of individuals, families, and the community. The terms welfare and well-being are often used interchangeably as well. Some people see welfare as primarily government-funded income support payments and welfare services. However, support and services in many areas of life aid welfare and are critical to the well-being of an individual and their family. The Organisation for Economic Co-operation and Development (OECD, 2015) states that well-being is multidimensional, covering aspects of life ranging from civic engagement to housing, from household income to work-life balance, and from skills to health status. A person's well-being is the result of risk, protective, and contextual factors. It can be influenced by social and economic factors at the individual, family, and community level, and each person's unique circumstances and experiences contribute to their well-being equation. Well-being can also influence, and be influenced by, a person's interaction with services and formal and informal supports. Determinants of well-being—or risk and protective factors—can positively or negatively affect a person's well-being and influence their need for welfare services and support. On an individual level, these factors include a person's circumstances, attitudes, behaviours, and how they respond to life events. On a broader scale, determinants affecting well-being include education, employment and skills, secure housing, social support networks, and health status. A person's economic well-being (i.e. income, consumption, and wealth) is a key determinant of their overall well-being as it influences greatly their ability to meet basic needs and maintain an acceptable standard of living.

9.2   Connecting Well-being and Health

Health, welfare, and well-being are strongly interrelated with the idea of "being well". The World Health Organization (WHO) defines health as "a state of complete physical, mental and social well-being and not merely the absence of disease and infirmity" (WHO, 1948), recognizing that one person's health status is linked to its well-being. Therefore, well-being is a multidimensional concept—as it was exposed previously—that has a direct impact on population health and could be easily devastated by situations that also affect people's health. Health is fundamental to an individual's well-being. Both physical and mental health such as chronic pain and stress are important aspects of health that affect well-being. A person's health status plays a role in their ability to participate in work, education, or training and engage with their community and social networks. Furthermore well-being is a sustainable condition that allows the individual or population to develop and thrive. The term subjective well-being is synonymous with positive mental health which could be potentially measured in terms of population health outcomes. In fact, the World Health Organization (WHO) defines positive mental health as "a state of well-being in which the individual realizes his or her own abilities, can cope with the normal stresses of life, can work productively and fruitfully, and is able to make a contribution to his or her community" (WHO, 2001). But this conceptualization of wellbeing goes beyond the absence of mental ill health, encompassing the perception that life is going well. Well-being has been linked to success at professional, personal, and interpersonal levels, with those individuals with a high level of well-being exhibiting greater productivity in the workplace, more effective learning, increased creativity, more prosocial behaviours, and positive relationships (Diener, 2012). In line with this, good health provides an individual with an ability to meet life's opportunities and challenges and maintain a level of functioning that has a positive influence on well-being.

Health is both a protective and a risk factor that can positively, or negatively, affect a person's well-being. For example, a person may suffer isolation or loneliness because of poor health. On the other hand, good health may enable them to earn a sufficient income to support themselves and live independently, placing them at lower risk of poor outcomes such as poor housing conditions, overcrowding, and homelessness. Conversely, the circumstances in which a person lives and works can affect their health. A number of social factors act together to strengthen or undermine health. These factors are also strongly related to well-being and include education, employment, social networks, social disadvantage, and lack of resources, opportunity, participation and skills, the built environment and location (McLachlan et al., 2013).

From this perspective, subjective well-being is a matter of positive experiences about various aspects of one's life, including the experiences of abundance, mental and physical health, progress, autonomy, self-acceptance, and relationships (Xing, 2013). Positive well-being is associated with being comfortable, happy, or healthy. It is not only good in itself, but has also been linked to many positive outcomes for mental and physical health, as well as improved interpersonal relationships and better community integration. For example, individuals with higher levels of subjective well-being have been shown to have stronger immune systems (Stone et al., 2018), to live longer (Ostir et al., 2000), to suffer from lower levels of sleep complaints (Brand et al., 2010), to exhibit greater self-control, self-regulatory and coping abilities (Fredrickson & Joiner, 2002), and to be relatively more cooperative, prosocial, charitable, and other-centred (Williams et al., 2018). Further, longitudinal data indicates that well-being in childhood goes on to predict future well-being in adulthood (Richards & Huppert, 2011) and higher well-being is linked to a number of better outcomes regarding physical health and longevity (Diener & Tov, 2012). Research on the connections between subjective well-being and physical health has drastically increased over the past twenty years, demonstrating a surge of interest in this topic. Overwhelmingly, subjective well-being is positively connected with physical health, revealing an impressive diversity of wellness benefits related to positive states and traits. To this end, one direction for future research is to determine whether overlapping constructs have separate effects on physical health. It is likely, however, that this literature is connected, since happy people tend to have more and better social relationships, and relationships confer well-being in many ways.

9.3 The Covid-19 Pandemic and Its Impact on Well-being and Health

The Coronavirus disease 2019 also known as Covid-19 is a major health threat caused by the SARS-CoV-2 virus, which has led to substantial disruption across almost all parts of society worldwide and consequently affecting well-being. Until the development of vaccines, the only practical way to contain its spread was by travel bans, strong physical distancing policies and practices, personal hygiene, closure of non-essential services, face masks, maintaining a minimum distance from others, strict quarantine and lockdown, strict isolation of cases and close contacts, establishing electronic check-in and QR codes to support contact tracing. The Covid-19 pandemic has direct effects on individuals who contract the virus, as well as many indirect effects on the broader community in terms of being well. These include changes to employment, income, living arrangements, and ability to spend time with friends and family. Whilst national governments spend substantial amounts of money collecting and analysing economic and, to a lesser extent, social and environmental indicators, relatively little attention has been given to how citizens actually experience their lives and especially in times of uncertainty such as in Covid-19 pandemic. In other words, much more is known about the material conditions of people's lives than about people's perceived quality of life, which we refer to as their well-being. However, those are the areas that have been mostly affected since the Covid-19 pandemic appeared worldwide.

The issue of the Covid-19 pandemic has occupied the agenda of the whole world since the beginning of 2020 to date. The pivot of this pandemic is a crucial element that has become almost as important as the virus itself, namely, the lockdown and its consequences such as the ones affecting the population well-being understood in terms of health outcomes. The Covid-19 pandemic has also highlighted the importance of our social relationships and connectedness. At the start of Covid-19, the restrictions to reduce the spread of the disease meant less social interactions for many people worldwide. The Organisation for Economic Co-operation and Development (OECD) has published data showing how the Covid-19 pandemic has hit all aspects of people's well-being in Europe and worldwide regarding health. Its report called *Covid-19 and well-being: life in the pandemic* (OECD, 2021a) says the virus caused a 16% increase in the average number of deaths across 33 OECD countries between March 2020 and early May 2021, compared with the same period over the previous four years. Over the same time frame, survey data in the report reveal rising levels of depression or anxiety and a growing sense among many people of loneliness and of feeling disconnected from society. The report says experiences of the pandemic have varied widely depending on age, gender, and ethnicity, as well as on the type of job people do and on their level of pay and skills. Mental health deteriorated for almost all population groups on average in 2020 but gaps in mental health by race and ethnicity are also visible. Covid-19 mortality rates for some ethnic minority communities have been more than twice those of other groups. Younger adults experienced some of the largest declines in mental health, social connectedness, and life satisfaction in 2020 and 2021, as well as facing job disruption and insecurity. Addressing the burden of poor physical and mental health and a cross-government approach to raising the well-being of the most disadvantaged children and youth must also be prioritized. The report in Europe (OECD, 2021b) focused on variables affecting health, quality of life, and well-being apart of mortality such as: risk of depression, risk of anxiety, very low life satisfaction, feeling lonely, feeling out of society, gaining weight, reducing exercise, increase of alcohol consumption, and start smoking. Moreover, in a paper examining the impact of Covid-19 on psychological health and well-being in the UK during a period of "lockdown" and the specific role of *Psychological Flexibility* as a potential mitigating process, high levels of distress were observed in the participating population (Dawson & Golijani-Moghaddam, 2020). However, psychological flexibility was significantly and positively associated with greater well-being, and inversely related to anxiety, depression, and Covid-19-related distress. Avoidant coping behaviour was positively associated with all indices of distress and negatively associated with well-being, while engagement in approach coping only demonstrated weaker associations with outcomes of interest. No relationship between adherence to government guidelines and psychological flexibility was found.

Continuing restrictions in place as result of the spread of the different variants of Covid-19 worldwide were likely to continue to impact people's feelings of social isolation and loneliness and have brought consequences nowadays. Although the rationale for lockdown is well-sustained by strong epidemiological arguments, exploring the barely unseen consequences of the contemporary Covid-19 pandemic from the perspective of health is mandatory for the consensus of a robust agreed position against numerous problems generated by the SARS-CoV-2 virus as well as preventing and early detecting future potentially similar situations. The SARS-CoV-2 virus has cut deeply into the fabric of our interconnectedness, to its own advantage, revealing the fragilities and vulnerabilities of our intertwined, complex social norms, values, systems, and functions. It has strained health systems, as well as social safety and emergency management architecture, also strongly affecting mobility around the world. Once again, we have learned that health is key for development, as a determinant of individual and collective growth, social cohesion, and resilience.

Health's central position in supporting the achievement of the United Nations Sustainable Development Goals, with its seven accelerator themes, especially during times of crisis, has proven that stronger intersectoral collaboration contributes to better health. Frontline health and essential social services workers have worked tirelessly and risked their lives in responding to the need for surge capacities. Health systems have been faced with ethical dilemmas on who can receive what type of care. Peer-to-peer, community-to-community, and country-to-country support have helped manage patient care. People's lives, with all their interlinkages and relationships, were severely disrupted as they were directed to stay physically apart to reduce infection. Billions of people were asked to stay at home; many lost their livelihoods and support networks. Children and young adults have been unable to continuously attend schools and universities, putting their well-being and future accomplishments at risk. Additionally, certain patients have demonstrated post-Covid conditions for a prolonged period of time. The mental health consequences of these disruptions have been severe, and a longer-term impact is expected. The Mental Health Coalition flagship initiative has been created and is more timely than ever. In some countries, the pandemic has revealed and exacerbated inequities and gaps that existed for people at the margins even before the virus arrived. The requirement to pay out of pocket for diagnostics and care during pandemics, and the lack of financial support packages to ensure livelihoods, has enlarged the circle of vulnerability and put humanity at risk. Such inequities demonstrate the importance of leaving no one behind and therefore initiatives should come from prevention, through testing, treatment, follow-up care and, where relevant, rehabilitation, and require universal access to comprehensive health care. It is time to take stock of the lessons learned so far, embrace new ways of thinking, and act swiftly to improve resilience in all levels of society, for this and for upcoming health emergencies.

9.4   Exploring the European Experience to Identify Good Practices and Lessons Learned

Starting from the rationale of the lockdown and the focus on the situation lived across Europe, in this chapter, we explore those consequences of the Covid-19 pandemic on the population well-being understood as health outcomes and specifically in the European context and allied countries. The good practices and lessons learned are still unknown to some extent for the scientific field that have emerged from the professional experience as the virus has spread faster than the production of scientific evidence. After this extensive but necessary introduction of the link between health and well-being, the aim of the rest of this chapter is to give voice to the health professionals' experiences and the organizations' initiatives in Europe and allied countries through the lessons they have learned in their day-to-day practice when facing population's well-being, in many cases shared with other colleagues in other parts of the world, and in others published in scientific journals by extracting those good practices on the basis of their experiential learning. A qualitative methodology approach based on a Delphi Technique was conducted with health professionals from different European regions considered as experts in highlighting the most prevalent health problems observed and solutions taken. The approach also shows the health outcomes mainly affected according to their lived experience and the good practices applied in their own professional settings to overcome the unknown and unexpected Covid-19 pandemic and improved positively the population well-being and health. The experts' reflections and feedback are supported by literature published regarding this topic and organizations' strate-gical positions. As we begin to think about recovery and "building back better", several key lessons to consider in moving forward have been identified from hands-on European informants considered as experts who lived the different pandemic waves in practice and had the responsibility to make decisions.

9.4.1   Mental Health and Covid-19: The Impact on Well-being and the Importance of Resilience

Health Professionals across Europe have pointed out that values such as equity, solidarity, and collaboration have been recognized since the first pandemic wave started by health practitioners as central to resilience and essential to drive an effective response, based around the concept that no one is safe until everyone is safe. Most of the professionals' discussions and publications point out the impor-tance of the professional values such as compassion, which seemed to have been forgotten in recent years. Populations have learned that one of the main principles of Preventive Medicine is to keep the others safe instead of not only oneself. Resilience against emergencies has become central to the United Nations Sustainable Devel-opment Goals and is a core principle of the World Health Organization European Programme of Work 2020–2025 (EPW) entitled "United Action for Better Health in Europe". Tailored support to countries and reinforcing regional preparedness and capacity to respond to emergencies are core priorities of the EPW. These are further strengthened by the EPW flagship initiatives, all of which have been at the forefront during Covid-19 pandemic: the Mental Health Coalition; Empowerment through Digital Health; the European Immunization Agenda 2030; and Healthier behaviours, incorporating behavioural and cultural insights. These initiatives correspond with the core areas identified by experts across Europe in this chapter and also by scientific publications.

The Covid-19 pandemic and government intervention such as lockdowns may have severely affected people's mental health. While lockdowns can help to contain the spread of the virus, they may result in substantial damage to population well-being. Brodeur et al. (2021) used Google Trends data to test whether Covid-19 and the associated lockdowns implemented in Europe and America led to changes in well-being using a related topic search-term and found a significant increase in searches for loneliness, worry, and sadness, while searches for stress, suicide, and divorce on the contrary fell. They also found a substantial increase in the search intensity for boredom in Europe and the US, what suggested that people's mental health may have been severely affected by the pandemic and lockdown. Some researchers have started discussing behavioural fatigue (Sibony, 2020) as individuals grow increasingly tired of self-regulating as time passes, which is an issue that is becoming more relevant with each wave of the pandemic. Behavioural fatigue, a little-known phrase not found in the most comprehensive textbook, has suddenly arisen to fame. The suggestion of experts is that people would get tired of staying at home so lockdown would be ineffective in the long term. This term could also be applied to those health professionals in practice that have been facing each wave. Moreover, Ammar et al. (2021) analysed the effects of home confinement on mental health and lifestyle behaviours during the Covid-19 outbreak and Covid-19 home confinement evoked a negative effect on mental well-being and emotional status with a greater proportion of individuals experiencing psychosocial and emotional disorders. These psychosocial tolls were associated with unhealthy lifestyle behaviours with a greater proportion of individuals experiencing physical and social inactivity, poor sleep quality, unhealthy diet behaviours, and unemployment. Conversely, participants demonstrated a greater use of technology during the confinement period. These findings elucidate the risk of psychosocial strain during the Covid-19 home confinement period and provide a clear remit for the urgent implementation of technology-based intervention to foster an active and healthy confinement lifestyle and also highlight the future population health problems.

Therefore, the Covid-19 pandemic has had a severe impact on the mental health and well-being of people around the world while also raising concerns of increased suicidal behaviour. In addition, access to mental health services has been severely impeded. However, no comprehensive summary of the current data on these impacts has until now been made widely available. A scientific brief (WHO, 2022) based on evidence from research commissioned by WHO, including an umbrella review of systematic reviews and meta-analyses and an update to a living systematic review provides a comprehensive overview of current evidence about:

- the impact of the Covid-19 pandemic on the prevalence of mental health symptoms and mental disorders which has increased worldwide.
- the impact of the Covid-19 pandemic on the prevalence of suicidal thoughts and behaviours which has increased worldwide too.
- the risk of infection, severe illness, and death from Covid-19 for people living with mental disorders which are higher.
- the impact of the Covid-19 pandemic on mental health services which requires more investment and new organization.
- the effectiveness of psychological interventions adapted to the Covid-19 pandemic to prevent or reduce mental health problems and/or maintain access to mental health services which seems to be working well.

Regarding mental health, European expert organizations and alliances such as the EU-Compass for Action on Mental Health and Well-being, the European Pact for Mental Health and Well-being among the member states, and the Pan-European Mental Health Coalition launched by the WHO, and the WHO European Framework for Action on Mental Health have stressed the importance of prioritizing resilience. Resilience is the ability of a system, community, or society, when exposed to hazards, to resist, absorb, accommodate, and recover in a timely and efficient manner, while retaining and restoring its essential basic structures and functions. Resilient infrastructures can shield societies by making systems more robust, keeping communities more connected, and keeping people healthier. Emergencies provide opportunities for deep systemic reviews and regular evaluations, followed by changes to build resilience, based on the lessons learned. The Covid-19 pandemic is therefore an opportunity to switch from bouncing back to bouncing forward, and from simply coping to anticipating and transforming, including through the introduction of digital tools where useful. Only when societies are well prepared and ready will responses become timelier and more effective, and will the adverse human, economic, and societal consequences of emergencies be significantly reduced and therefore the populations' well-being becomes improved.

9.4.2 Healthcare Professionals' Well-being and their Coping Strategies

From the perspective of the Healthcare Providers' well-being most of the publications relate to mental health and psychological effects and specifically with stress, anxiety, resilience, and coping. Working under pandemic conditions exposes health care workers not only to infection risk but also to psychological strain and this is something lived by in all the European professionals and health organizations. The article published in 2022 about the experience of European hospital-based health care workers on following infection prevention and control procedures and their well-being during the first wave of the Covid-19 pandemic (Van Hout et al., 2022) conducted in 40 European countries mainly with medical doctors and nurses directly treating patients with Covid-19 reported they were fearful of caring for these patients, having high levels of concern about Covid-19 infection risk to themselves and their family as a result of their job and considered that getting infected with Covid-19 was not within their control especially among junior staff.

Much has been written especially about nurses in the health professional literature in the last years due to their frontline positions during the pandemic situation and especially those from intensive care units, emergency rooms, and inpatient hospitalization units, apart from the fact that 2020 was declared by the World Health Organization as the Year of the Nurses and Midwives. Media has pointed to the nursing profession as one of the professions which has been most negatively affected by Covid-19. Professionals' reflections about caring for patients with Covid-19 and their lived experience to the concept of resilience are the common issue in most of the articles published by the majority of journals and is one of the highly mentioned effects of the pandemic situation by professionals across Europe. Thusini (2020) discussed the similarities and differences to pre-pandemic understandings of resilience and factors that usually mediate acute stress, resilience, and psychological recovery during a pandemic. The resources to support nurses and other healthcare staff to manage stress and promote well-being are important research directions that warrant attention. The stories published using qualitative methods are ones of learning and hope and, importantly, they capture key lessons that could equip healthcare staff with positive coping strategies in a time of unprecedented pressure worldwide and specifically in European societies and health systems based on welfare. Furthermore, destigmatizing mental health is necessary for healthcare providers to empower them to seek support and has been a central issue as was highlighted by Shah et al. (2021). These authors recommended that hospital administrators should develop proactive wellness plans for the triage and management of mental and emotional health needs during a pandemic that prioritizes transparent communication, resources for healthcare providers within and beyond the clinical setting and training. Experts from different European regions have reiterated that the Covid-19 pandemic is placing unprecedented pressure on nurses and other health professional workforce that is already under considerable mental strain due to overloaded systems. Convergent evidence from the pandemics indicates that nurses experience the highest levels of psychological distress compared with other health professionals. In line with this, nurse leaders are facing particular challenges in mitigating risk and supporting nursing staff to negotiate moral distress and fatigue during large-scale, sustained crises. Synthesizing the burgeoning literature on Covid-19-related burnout and moral distress faced by nurses and identifying effective interventions to reduce poor mental health outcomes will enable nurse leaders to support the resilience of their teams (Sriharan et al., 2021).

Apart from the directly and indirectly well-being-based training disseminated by WHO for professional staff since the Covid pandemic started, a brief commissioned by the International Centre for Nurse Migration (ICNM) and the International Council of Nurses (ICN) in 2022 provides a global snapshot assessment of how the Covid-19 pandemic is impacting on the nursing workforce (Buchan et al., 2022), with a specific focus on how changing patterns of nurse supply and mobility will challenge the sustainability of the global nursing workforce which is nowadays experiencing important shortages worldwide though especially in the high-income countries. It also sets out the urgent action agenda and global workforce plan for 2022 and beyond which is required to support nurse workforce sustainability, and therefore improve health system responsiveness and resilience in the face of Covid-19. To mitigate these damaging effects, and to improve longer-term nurse workforce sustainability, there is an urgent need for effective and coordinated policy responses both at national level and internationally. This response must include both immediate action to meet the urgent challenges set out in the brief and the development of a shared longer-term vision and plan for the global nursing workforce, to ensure that the world is better placed in the future to meet major health shocks.

The following is required:

- At country level:
  - Commitment to support for safe staffing levels based on consistent application of staffing methods, necessary resource allocation, and health system good governance
  - Commitment to support for early access to full vaccinations programmes for all nurses; no matter whether they practice either in public or private systems

- Nurse workforce impact assessments, conducted regularly in order to generate evidence and develop a better understanding of the impact of the pandemic on individual nurses and the overall nursing workforce
- Reviewing and expanding the capacity of the domestic nurse education system which should be based on data generated from impact assessments and from a regular and systematic national nurse labour market analysis
- Assessing and improving retention of nurses and the attractiveness of nursing as a career, by ensuring that the damaging effect of Covid-19 burnout of nurses is addressed, and by the provision of fair pay and conditions of employment, structured career opportunities, and access to continuing education;
- Implementing policies to enable the nursing workforce's contribution to pandemic response to be optimized through supporting advanced practice and specialist roles, effective skill mix and working patterns, teamworking, and provision of appropriate technology and equipment, as well as training in its use
- Monitoring and tracking nurse self-sufficiency by using the self-sufficiency indicator of level of reliance on foreign-born or foreign-trained nurses

• At international level, key stakeholders should start acting from now on, and also develop and agree on a vision and long-term plan for sustaining the global nursing workforce that is highly in risk by:

- Supporting an immediate update of the State of the World's Nursing (SOWN) analysis. As we entered the third year of the pandemic, there was an urgent need for an updated global profile of the nursing workforce to assess the damage done and the scope for targeted action on sustainability and renewal
- Commitment to support for early access to full vaccinations programmes for all nurses, in all countries. International cooperation is required to protect the nursing workforce in all countries, no matter the nation they belong to
- Commitment to implementing and evaluating effective and ethical approaches to managed international supply of nurses, through a collective approach framed within a fuller implementation of the WHO Global Code of Practice on the International Recruitment of Health Personnel. This must focus on improved monitoring of international flows of nurses, independent monitoring of the use of country-to-country bilateral agreements and recruitment agencies to ensure compliance, and with fair and transparent recruitment and employment practices
- Commitment to supporting regular and systematic nurse workforce impact assessments, particularly in resource constrained countries, by the provision of technical advice, data improvement, independent analysis, and multi-stakeholder policy dialogues to agree priority policy actions on domestic nurse supply and retention
- Commitment to investing in nurse workforce sustainability in small states, lower-income states, and fragile states, most vulnerable to nurse outflow, and impacted by the pandemic, by building on the lessons of the United Nations High Level Commission on Health Employment and Economic Growth, and

of the WHO Strategic Directions on Nursing and Midwifery which demonstrate the long-term economic, social, and population health benefits of investing in the nursing workforce

- There is also need for both urgent action and a shared long-term vision and plan for the global nursing workforce. The Covid-19 pandemic has caused unprecedented damage to the global nursing workforce and is already creating additional harm in 2022. Without sufficient well motivated and supported nurses, the global health system cannot function.
- It is urgently needed to meet internationally the 2022 Action Agenda and to develop a longer-term plan to improve nurse retention and give hope for the future sustainability of the profession.

A case of good practice aligned with all these aspects and requirements is the ProCare European Commission funded project whose overall aim has been along the Covid-19 pandemic to enhance the research alliance between partner hospitals and HEIs, one gap that already existed from before, to raise the profile of research in nursing and thus improve patient outcomes. This project has aimed also to encourage such alliances across Europe via a freely available online learning programme and a guidance document on developing nursing research as example of good practice of the knowledge triangle implementation in nursing research development. ProCare's mission is not to educate future nursing researchers but to train the nursing workforce in practice to use the scientific evidence coming from research in a beneficial way so that it impacts positively on populations' health outcomes.

Students' mental well-being as future professionals is of critical importance as well. Even though data on medical students' mental health during Covid-19 are scarce and have been somewhat conflicting, early detection and intervention strategies should be implemented in order to help future physicians, nurses, and other health professionals go through this challenging period and be better prepared for next large-scale crises. A large systematic review and meta-analysis of 129,123 medical students in 47 countries, including European ones, conducted pre-Covid-19 estimated that the prevalence of depression or depressive symptoms was 27.2% and the overall pooled crude prevalence of suicidal ideation was 11.1% (Rotenstein et al., 2016). According to European experts those results have got worse as the pandemic waves have appeared and have also been associated in students from the field of health with high levels of anxiety and panic, sleep quality appears to have deteriorated during the pandemic, with insomnia, difficulties falling asleep, and frequent awakening during the night as well as decreased appetite.

9.4.3 Healthcare Policies, Human Rights Affecting Well-being and Universal Healthcare Coverage

In the paper published by Burlacu et al. (2020) the other consequences of the Covid-19 pandemic measures were explored and exposed such as the use or abuse of human rights and freedom restrictions, economic issues, marginalized groups, and eclipse of all other diseases in Europe. Their scientific attempt is to coagulate a stable position and integrate current opposing views by advancing the idea that rather than applying the uniform lockdown policy, one could recommend instead an improved model targeting stricter and more prolonged lockdowns to vulnerable risk/age groups while enabling less stringent measures for the lower-risk groups, minimizing both economic losses and deaths. Rigorous (and also governed by freedom) debating may be able to synchronize the opposed perspectives between those advocating an extreme lockdown (e.g. most of the epidemiologists and health experts) and those criticizing all restrictive measures (e.g. economists, anti-vaccination groups, and human rights experts). Confronting the multiple facets of the public health mitigation measures is the only way to avoid contributing to history with yet another failure, as seen in other past epidemics.

Worldwide, the social protection programmes have become a key tool for policymakers. These programmes are executed to achieve multiple objectives such as fighting poverty and hunger and increasing the resilience of the poor and vulnerable groups towards various shocks. In fact, with the rapid spread of the Covid-19 pandemic, many countries started to implement social protection programmes to eliminate the negative impacts of the Covid-19 pandemic crisis and enhance community resilience. The European Pillar of Social Rights (EPSR) Action Plan published by the European Commission in 2021 draws attention to the significant impact of Covid-19 on jobs and welfare systems across Europe, and consequently directly and indirectly affecting population health (Urquijo, 2021). In its Porto Declaration (2021), the European Council recognizes such challenges and underlines the EU commitment to continue deepening the implementation of the EPSR at EU and national levels, establishing among its key priorities: the need to reduce inequalities, defend fair wages, fight social exclusion and tackle poverty, promote equality and fairness, support young people and address the risks of exclusion for particularly vulnerable social groups (Baptista et al., 2021). This report examines the national social protection and inclusion policy measures that European countries put in place to help address the social and financial distress created by the pandemic and by lockdown policies. It covers the 27 EU Member States, the 7 candidate and potential candidate countries, and the UK. It reveals an overall rapid reaction through the introduction of mostly temporary measures—primarily relaxing eligibility conditions, increasing benefit levels, and creating new ad hoc social and job protection schemes. These emergency measures helped avert a massive social crisis and some would have seemed impossible one year previously. Yet they also highlighted weaknesses and gaps in existing social protection and inclusion policies, and the pressing need to address these. Although these measures were the main tools used to tackle the socio-economic impact of the pandemic, the report underlines their limited transformative potential for countries' social protection systems. The report proposes a series of specific actions that could usefully be considered at national and/or EU level.

UNICEF's Evaluation Office and Programme Division jointly commissioned the Economic Policy Research Institute (EPRI) to conduct a rapid review of social protection responses to the Covid-19 pandemic. In relation to Europe, the country brief presents the initial findings of the rapid review of Montenegro's social protection response to the crisis (UNICEF, 2021). Montenegro was the Western Balkans' fastest developing economy prior to the pandemic. The review is based on desk research, interviews with eight key informants, a validation webinar with UNICEF country representatives, and interaction with 19 other country case studies. The review highlights that in some small European countries with limited capacity in the health sector (lack of human resources, weak health structures, and limited availability of medical supplies to cover the entire population) support from donors and development organizations proved crucial. Adaptation, however, proved challenging given the constraints of the necessary public health response. Adaptation of the pre-existing social protection was essential in targeting the "new poor" and the already vulnerable sections existing pre-Covid-19. In Montenegro, new social protection interventions targeting the newly vulnerable proved significantly more challenging due to the means-tested eligibility criteria. Governments should look to strengthen service delivery capacity, especially sustainable implementation of activation programmes in the labour market. Work activation programmes such as providing information, counselling, and motivation services, active employment policy programmes and employment mediation help develop individual capacity and increase their access to the labour market. It is important to ensure that the opportunities available to the working-age population are financially adequate and respond to the needs of the unemployed population.

Experts recommend to anchor all actions in a trusted social contract. Equity, solidarity, and responsiveness must be the basis of actions to improve health, social, and educational services with financial protection. Thus, a national health architecture anchored in all levels of government must encourage participation, be sensitive to cultural norms, and be responsive to the individual's needs, with particular attention to vulnerable groups that can differ depending on the context and type of emergency crisis. Safeguarding such an intricate and interconnected health and social system requires strong governance structures, clear sets of national priorities, and plans for health emergency readiness that are included in all policies across different sectors.

Another recommendation that came up from experts' discussion has to do with integrating emergency public health services and universal health coverage. Countries with universal health coverage based on strong public health and primary health care services were more agile, adaptable, and ready to deliver a comprehensive response to the pandemic. The experience of these countries can serve as a model for how to provide continuous and quality dual-track (emergency-related and routine) services, help people avoid out-of-pocket payments, repurpose a digital health information system to implement basic response measures (such as testing, tracing, and isolating or quarantining), and integrate core health programmes such as those on mental health into emergency management.

9.4.4 New Learning Opportunities and the Boost of Digital and Technological Development

Governance of data and digital technology use is a key lesson learned from the pandemic. It has been demonstrated that it is necessary to establish and update digital health platforms. Having well-articulated principles, standards, and governance of data and digital technologies during pandemics and other health emergencies is vital to ensure that trust is established in their use and, in turn, for the delivery of an effective and proportionate public health response. Accountability and oversight mechanisms need to be included as part of good governance, in addition to the monitoring and evaluation of the public health impact. The role of publicly owned digital platforms should be strengthened to ensure public trust in and security of public data.

In fact, Covid-19 has had a crippling effect on the health care systems around the world with cancellation of elective medical services and disruption of daily life. Experts and authors such as Iyengar et al. (2020) have highlighted the learning opportunities offered by the pandemic and their implication for a better future health care system through a comprehensive review of the current literature undertaken to analyse the consequences of Covid-19 on health care systems by using suitable keywords like "Covid-19", "telemedicine", "health care", and "remote consultations" on the search engines of PubMed, SCOPUS, Google Scholar, and Research Gate. There has been a shared drive worldwide to devise strategies to protect people against viral transmission with reinforcement of hand hygiene and infection control principles but also to provide continuity of health care. Virtual and remote technologies have been increasingly used in health care management. Covid-19 has offered unique learning opportunities for the health care sector. Yet, according to Age Platform Europe (2021) this fast digitalization is also pushing aside a growing number of people in preventing them to access essential services, as many older people's organizations across Europe have warned (Kucharczyk, 2021). Members of the Age Platform Europe have reported different though similar situations across Europe. In fact, The Flemish Council of the Elderly warns against a widening gap between those who are digitally active and the growing group of people who are unable to do so or for whom it goes too fast. In fact, 1 out of 4 survey respondents indicated that they do not feel comfortable with the sudden change to more digital and online applications. Remarkably, this is even the case for 30% of young people and the over-65 s. Although the majority of the Flemish population has a positive attitude vis-à-vis technology, they are wrestling with a number of paradoxes: the advantages of online tools versus the dependency on their smartphone and social media, the availability of a wide range of news sources versus the dangers of disinformation, the ease of use of data-driven services versus the concern for our privacy, security, and control over their personal data. In the Netherlands, a survey carried out by the older people organization KBO-PCOB finds that many older people do not want to be obliged on the Internet. Nine out of ten Internet-free (91%) and half (46%) of the online seniors agree are tired of being forced to do everything over the Internet. Almost all of them (98% offline senior, 94% online senior) think that companies and governments should always offer an alternative for people without the Internet. In Spain, UDP Mayores reports the findings of the 2nd "Covid Social Services Impact Monitor Report" and highlighted the digital divide, loneliness, and social isolation of many older people as one of the biggest challenges facing institutions. To address the digital divide, improving digital literacy is key according to experts. Age Platform Europe members are providing digital training classes and materials. Such is the case of: Eläkeliiton (Finland) that has been involved in a number of projects, activities, and materials intended for media education professionals and older people; Old'Up (France) has produced a training guide to help informal and professional carers train older people in using digital tablet; the Digital Compass (Germany) is a network of 75 Internet pilot support locations where older people can meet and try out digital services. In Greece, 50+ Hellas shares on its website digital educational material. The organization also joined the "Knowledge Volunteers" project which organized digital trainings of older adults thanks to the recruitment of young volunteers. In Spain, UDP Mayores is organizing basic digital classes for its members. The Spanish Confederation of Older People's Organisations CEOMA also organizes a cycle of webinars on teaching how to use technological tools to help reduce isolation and loneliness.

Rationalizing and optimizing available resources with resilience shown on the coronavirus frontline during the crisis are some of most important lessons learnt during the crisis. Importance of personal hygiene and reinforcement of infection control measures have been acknowledged. Telemedicine revolution will be a vital factor in delivering health care in the future though from an inclusive perspective and trying not to leave anyone out. Investing in health care infrastructure and workforce was another theme that emerged from experts' contributions. Increased training for and material support to frontline health workers must be provided alongside new mechanisms for activating required surge capacity, including countries' knowledge and their readiness to receive and send external support. Additional workforce for emergencies, including volunteers and those from civil society organizations, should be trained in advance to support emerging needs in real time. Investing in the emergency and dual service health care workforce would allow for the continuity of all health and social services during emergencies.

Transforming scientific discoveries into accessible public health goods that are affordable remains urgent according to the lived experience. The collaboration demonstrated by the global scientific community in isolating and sequencing SARS-CoV-2 within the first 10 days of 2020, and delivering a vaccine from bench to bedside within the subsequent 12 months, while adhering to the highest quality standards, was unprecedented and exemplifies the rapidly evolving break-throughs emerging in biotechnology, genetics and epidemiology in particular, and in health care and medicine in general. Going forward, further investment in early identification, diagnostics, new medicines development and the repurposing of existing ones, vaccination technologies, sharing know-how, and ensuring equitable and scalable access for all are the necessary next steps in building on these historic achievements and turning them into a global public health good. In line with this, leveraging health information for immediate and robust action is crucial. The role that health and social data collection, analyses and distribution can play in driving decision-making has been long underestimated, and such data have therefore been underutilized. Data sets rapidly shared across health care and civic institutions, both within domestic borders and beyond, enabled practical and responsible Covid-related policy-making. However, the true life-saving potential of leveraging troves of data and common definitions and key indicators has yet to be uncovered. Building the resilience of health systems to future pandemics requires a paradigm shift in how health and health-related data are sourced, governed, accessed, certified, assessed, protected, and shared.

The "One Health" approach in collecting multisectoral data can serve as a model in this regard. As per the definition provided by the One Health Initiative Task Force, One Health implies "the collaborative efforts of multiple disciplines working locally, nationally, and globally, to attain optimal health for people, animals and our environment" (American Veterinary Medical Association, 2008). In other and simpler words, "you cannot tell the story of human health separate from animal health or environmental health". The One Health European Joint Programme (OHEJP) aims at creating a sustainable European framework by integration and alignment of medical, veterinary, and food institutes through joint programming of research agendas matching the needs of European and national policymakers and stakeholders. OHEJP in line with the "Prevent-Detect-Respond" concept is focused on reinforcing collaboration between institutes by enhancing transdisciplinary cooperation and integration of activities by means of dedicated Joint Research Projects, Joint Integrative Project and through education and training in the fields of Foodborne Zoonoses, Antimicrobial Resistance, and Emerging Threats. Through the OHEJP there are opportunities for harmonization of approaches, methodologies, databases, and procedures for the assessment and management of foodborne hazards, emerging threats, and AMR across Europe, which will improve the quality and compatibility of information for decision-making. The Joint Research Projects and Joint Integrative Projects are key instruments to facilitate partner organizations working together and aligning their approaches, increasing their knowledge base of host–microbe interactions, and improving epidemiological studies and risk assessments which ultimately equip risk managers with the best tools for intervention measures.

Accordingly, it is important to prioritize known capacity gaps. While existing international frameworks are a powerful operational backbone, many member states in the region did not seek or utilize potential collaborations to the full. The pandemic has highlighted the strengths of many aspects of the International Health Regulations (IHR) (2005) and instruments such as the Cartagena Protocol on Biosafety, and the Nagoya Protocol on Access to Genetic Resources and the Fair and Equitable Sharing of Benefits Arising from their Utilization to the Convention on Biological Diversity. It has validated the importance of preparedness efforts towards combating pandemic influenza by implementing lessons learned from previous outbreaks (e.g. Ebola, SARS, MERS-CoV, and Zika). However, there is more work to be done. As countries seek to equip themselves with tools to withstand health emergencies at all levels of society, we must address the gaps identified in the IHR (2005) and in existing frameworks and pursue a diversified portfolio of whole-of-government and whole-of-society preparedness and response.

Furthermore, the current epidemic situation has made every higher education institution (HEI) acutely aware of the need to create blended/distance learning courses. It is vital that these are created in a way that optimizes learning and ensures the students' further development of their skills and competences in the future. Simulation which is a core part of the future health professionals' training seems to be a safe way to train healthcare providers to provide effective care for older people and their families when it is conducted online and digitally. There is evidence that simulation-training can improve the quality of care provided for older people. High-fidelity simulation could therefore become a good solution to overcome the lack of mobility in Europe for the future health professionals. However, although geriatric simulation programmes are being undertaken worldwide, hardly any touches on the issue of intercultural differences as a problem that professional geriatric nurses should be well conscious of and less or even none are based on high fidelity. In this context, the objectives of GNurseSIM, a European Commission funded Project under Erasmus+ are to support HEI to provide students in geriatric nursing with opportunities during their training to practise skills of adopting a multidisciplinary holistic approach to the care of older patients throughout the High-Fidelity Simulation approach. This will be achieved by combining elements from different approaches to arrive at a unified model and develop an intercultural, culture-sensitive geriatric nursing course, as well as recommendations and guidelines regarding the implementation of the course and possibilities it offers to other areas of nursing.

Moreover, another case of good practice to be pointed out are HEALINT and HEALINT4ALL Projects, both of them supported by the European Commission, whose aim is to support students from the field of health in participating in best practice environments. They start from the rationale that quality processes must be in place and these require innovation to assure audit material resources that are fit for purpose, can work well within the situation, and provide the correct teaching and learning to train auditors. Quality assured clinical learning, including evidence shared across boundaries, will support a globally prepared medical international workforce able to transfer skills and practice and offer best interventions to enhance patient treatment throughout digital development. Shared evidence is essential within the EU, due to benefits of free movement, of health professionals across borders and cross border healthcare, which includes movement of patients to receive treatment. Such perspective includes requirements to ensure parity of competence and standards of professional proficiency, and their very presence points to the necessity of cultural appreciation and understanding of the needs of patients across borders. HEALINT and HEALINT4ALL are focused on providing Medical Education and Professionals Allied to Medicine a digital interactive audit system to facilitate quality assurance of EU clinical learning environments so that European Healthcare students will be confident that they can obtain an increased number and variety of safe optimized learning placements through extensive partnerships developed, thus fostering inclusivity.

9.4.5 The Interconnectedness of Health Systems and Emergency Preparedness

Health systems must be placed at the centre of national agendas, while emergency preparedness needs to be at the core of all health systems' functions. The resilience and preparedness of health systems and related organizations are necessary preconditions to building wider resilience against health emergencies, but neither is sufficient alone. In the future, to avoid crippling effects such as those that Covid-19 has had on our societies, this dual relationship must be reflected and implemented in national agendas. It is important to recognize that health emergencies impact the whole of society, including its socio-economic systems, investments in preparedness and mitigation measures for improving essential public health functions and primary and hospital services yield long-term dividends, directly saving lives and preventing human suffering, while protecting the economy and fostering trust in governments in times of vulnerability.

It is essential to ensure that response systems are functional long before emergencies strike. All-hazards emergency prevention and preparedness activities have proven to be critical for a swift, comprehensive response. Having a functional response frameworks and systems prior to the pandemic enabled countries to achieve better organized and coordinated action. Individual technical public health and IHR (2005) core capacities (laboratory, surveillance, etc.), even when monitored and evaluated (including through simulation exercises, voluntary peer reviews, after-action reviews, and State Party Annual Reporting), did not fully represent the needed emergency preparedness and readiness. To improve preparedness and response, IHR (2005) core capacities need to be fortified by capabilities and competencies at all levels of governance, by services and by communities.

In the context of Covid-19, the response early on in the pandemic was slower than the spread of the virus and therefore this fact showed that health systems and emergency coordination were not as interconnected and steady as it was supposed. This situation makes us think of the continuing professional development (CPD) which could be core for the interconnectedness of health systems and emergency preparedness as well as an essential tool for healthcare professionals to deliver high-quality and safe person-centred care, amidst ever-changing health systems across the globe and especially in situations such as pandemics. The World Health Organization (WHO) cited a skilled workforce as the cornerstone of a healthy nation and supported the need to expand transformative, high-quality education and life-long learning for all healthcare workers (WHO, 2016). A coordinated approach is needed to determine how CPD programmes and activities can address workforce planning and the recruitment and retention of healthcare workers and other workers in the health systems. This approach supports strategies to confront the current global recruitment and retention crisis of healthcare workers to achieve a quality healthcare system for all people. Evaluation of CPD activities is an essential part of the programme measuring whether and to what extent they improve the delivery of high-quality, safe person-centred care. CPD activities should be able to demonstrate the sustainability and efficiency of the programme. However there is limited data on the economic cost of training health professionals and very little is known about the economic cost and cost-effectiveness of providing CPD to healthcare professionals, according to the scoping review conducted by Orlik et al. (2022) the research working group team of the European Centre of Excellence for Research in CPD at the Royal College of Surgeons in Ireland. The authors of this review emphasize the need to standardize the methods applied in CPD programmes as well as the need of evidence and proof of the return on investments. It is understood that such a process of standardization requires time, and researchers should be encouraged to identify experts with skills and knowledge in economic evaluations, particularly regarding the design and implementation of CPD programmes. This standardization is of importance in times of healthcare expenditure cuts and increasing demand in the prioritized allocation of funds in healthcare spending such as ageing populations, global demographic growth, and more recently the emergence of Covid-19. Economic evaluations can provide useful information to those making decisions about the allocation of limited health care resources. In particular, economic evaluations can be used to identify interventions that are vital to the health service (health professionals, organizations, and patients) and those that provide little benefit given the resources required. The ultimate test of an economic evaluation is whether it leads to better decisions in the presence of uncertainty and results in the more efficient and effective use of limited healthcare resources. There is an important role for economic evaluations in priority setting in health care decision-making. This includes assessing the cost-effectiveness of CPD activities for healthcare professionals. Consequently, an economic evaluation of CPD activities can be used to maximize the benefits from health care spending in this area and to contain costs and manage the needs of the health service. In line with this the European Centre of Excellence for Research in Continuing Professional Development aims to establish a pan-European network of researchers, clinicians, regulators, and professional bodies to advance the science of continuing professional development (CPD) through research, fostering partnerships that enable knowledge exchange to attain CPD best practices across Europe with the focus on three critical goals:

- To support collaborative research projects among European and national partners.
- To build networks among academic and clinical practice colleagues and organizations to boost CPD research.
- To develop and strengthen national CPD systems in European countries through data-driven knowledge about CPD best practice.

9.4.6   Challenges of Covid-19 for Professional Development and Opportunities for the Future

Covid-19 pandemic has undoubtedly disrupted the well-established, traditional structure of health systems, welfare systems, and health workforce across Europe impacting negatively on populations' well-being. The new limitations of physical presence have accelerated the development of online learning environments for different sorts of communication such as telemedicine consultation, comprising both asynchronous and synchronous distance communication and education, and the introduction of novel ways of patients' and students' assessment. At the same time, this prolonged crisis has had serious implications on the lives of individuals including their psychological well-being and the impact on their social trajectories. The new reality has, on many occasions, triggered the "acting up" of health professions' workers and students as frontline healthcare staff, which has been perceived by many of them as a positive or negative learning and contributing experience, and has led to a variety of responses from the institutions. The need for substitution of the daily live and hands-on education during this pandemic has cultivated the incorporation of a variety of innovational ideas into medical education across Europe, which have involved the introduction of new technological concepts, and also novel ways for medical educators to interact with their students. All these innovative methods should be carefully examined, as they could constitute a source of future inspiration for medical educators. These encompass social media initiatives, virtual core clerkships and digital clinical placements, new teaching models, sessions of remote patient consultation, even the use of patient simulators.

There is no need to stress the importance of health professional specialities such as those related with Preventive Medicine and Vaccinology nowadays. Furthermore, Hayden and Parkin (2020) stated that Pharmacists, like psychiatrists, have modified their practices amidst Covid-19 in order to guarantee care and support to their patients. Designated essential frontline services and community pharmacists are facing a spectrum of challenges to surmount to ensure patient care continues. These include assisting in the prevention of infection, managing supply chains, preventing stockpiling, and provision of evidence-based medical information. However, disasters like Covid-19 disproportionately affect poor and vulnerable populations, and patients with mental health conditions may be among the hardest hit. Pharmacist-level, system-level, and regulatory responses have sought to minimize this impact, although there is likely to be a lasting impact on the profession, both good and bad. Another recommendation for professional support and role expansion is the case of mental health Nursing and Community Nursing. A similar situation is the one lived by Nurse Prescribing as a professional competency that had been discussed in different European countries for years though nowadays experts remark as a crucial support to monitor chronic patients, among others, that would have been necessary during the critical periods of each pandemic wave. NUPHAC (Nurse and Pharmaceutical Care) is a European network that aims at strengthening evidence, policy, practice, and education in nurses' contribution to interprofessional pharmaceutical care in relation with the European Pharmaceutical Strategy. NUPHAC have stressed the fact that nurses are insufficiently represented in pharmaceutical care related debates and the Covid-19 pandemic has highlighted a lot of potential to improve quality of care through interprofessional collaboration in pharmaceutical care across Europe. Other fields that are gaining momentum nowadays are Biomedical Engineers, Robotics, Artificial Intelligence, and others related with the new paradigm. The OECD report in 2021 regarding the Covid pandemic says reinforcing trust is key to reconnecting people to their societies, and to the institutions that are meant to support them. By doing so, the well-being of citizens will be improved both today and in a post-pandemic future.

References

American Veterinary Medical Association. (2008). *One health: A new professional imperative*. One Health Initiative Task Force: Final Report, 15.

Ammar, A., Trabelsi, K., Brach, M., Chtourou, H., Boukhris, O., Masmoudi, L., Bouaziz, B., Bentlage, E., How, D., Ahmed, M., Mueller, P., Mueller, N., Hammouda, O., Paineiras-Domingos, L. L., Braakman-Jansen, A., Wrede, C., Bastoni, S., Pernambuco, C. S., Mataruna, L., Taheri, M., et al. (2021). Effects of home confinement on mental health and lifestyle behaviours during the COVID-19 outbreak: Insights from the ECLB-COVID19 multicentre study. *Biology of Sport, 38*(1), 9–21.

Baptista, I., Marlier, E., Spasova, S., Peña-Casas, R., Fronteddu, B., Ghailani, D., Sabato, S., & Regazzoni, P. (2021). *Social protection and inclusion policy responses to the COVID-19 crisis. An analysis of policies in 35 countries*. European Social Policy Network (ESPN).

Brand, S., Gerber, M., Beck, J., Hatzinger, M., Pühse, U. W. E., & Holsboer-Trachsler, E. (2010). Exercising, sleep-EEG patterns, and psychological functioning are related among adolescents. *The World Journal of Biological Psychiatry, 11*(2), 129–140.

Brodeur, A., Clark, A. E., Fleche, S., & Powdthavee, N. (2021). COVID-19, lockdowns and well-being: Evidence from Google trends. *Journal of Public Economics, 193*, 104346.

Buchan, J., Catton, H., & Shaffer, F. (2022). Sustain and retain in 2022 and beyond. *International Council of Nurses, 71*, 1–71.

Burlacu, A., Crisan-Dabija, R., Covic, A., Raiu, C., Mavrichi, I., Popa, I. V., & Lillo-Crespo, M. (2020). Pandemic lockdown, healthcare policies and human rights: Integrating opposed views on Covid-19 public health mitigation measures. *Reviews in Cardiovascular Medicine, 21*(4), 509–516.

Dawson, D. L., & Golijani-Moghaddam, N. (2020). Covid-19: Psychological flexibility, coping, mental health, and well-being in the UK during the pandemic. *Journal of Contextual Behavioral Science, 17*, 126–134.

Diener, E. (2012). New findings and future directions for subjective well-being research. *American Psychologist, 67*(8), 590.

Diener, E., Lucas, R. E., Kahneman, D., & Schwarz, N. (1999). 11 personality and subjective well-being. *Ell-being: Foundations of Hedonic Psychology, 213*, 1.

Diener, E., & Tov, W. (2012). *National accounts of well-being (Handbook of social indicators and quality of life research)* (pp. 137–157). Springer.

European Commission. (2021). *European Pillar of Social Rights (EPSR) action plan*.

European Council. (2021). *Porto declaration*.

Fredrickson, B. L., & Joiner, T. (2002). Positive emotions trigger upward spirals toward emotional well-being. *Psychological Science, 13*(2), 172–175.

Hayden, J. C., & Parkin, R. (2020). The challenges of COVID-19 for community pharmacists and opportunities for the future. *Irish Journal of Psychological Medicine, 37*(3), 198–203.

Hefferon, K., & Boniwell, I. (2011). *Positive psychology.* OpenUniversity Press.

Huppert, F. A., Marks, N., Clark, A., Siegrist, J., Stutzer, A., Vittersø, J., & Wahrendorf, M. (2009). Measuring well-being across Europe: Description of the ESS well-being module and preliminary findings. *Social Indicators Research, 91*(3), 301–315.

Huta, V., & Ryan, R. M. (2010). Pursuing pleasure or virtue: The differential and overlapping well-being benefits of hedonic and eudaimonic motives. *Journal of Happiness Studies, 11*(6), 735–762.

Iyengar, K., Mabrouk, A., Jain, V. K., Venkatesan, A., & Vaishya, R. (2020). Learning opportunities from COVID-19 and future effects on health care system. *Diabetes and Metabolic Syndrome: Clinical Research and Reviews, 14*(5), 943–946.

Kashdan, T. B., Biswas-Diener, R., & King, L. (2008). Reconsidering happiness: The costs of distinguishing between hedonics and eudaimonia. *The Journal of Positive Psychology, 3*(4), 219–233. https://doi.org/10.1080/17439760802303044

Keyes, C. L. M., Shmotkin, D., & Ryff, C. D. (2002). Optimizing well-being: The empirical encounter of two traditions. *Journal of Personality and Social Psychology, 82*(6), 1007–1022.

Kucharczyk, M. (2021). *Towards an EU age equality strategy: Delivering equal rights at all ages.* AGE Platform Europe.

McLachlan, R., Gilfillan, G., & Gordon, J. (2013). *Deep and persistent disadvantage in Australia.* Productivity Commission.

OECD. (2021a). *Covid-19 and well-being: Life in the Pandemic publication.* www.oecd.org/wise/Covid-19-and-well-being-1e1ecb53-en.htm.

OECD. (2021b). *Covid-19 well-being country notes data publication.* www.oecd.org/wise/COVID-19-well-being-country-notes-data.xlsx.

OECD (Organisation for Economic Co-operation and Development). (2015). *How's life? 2015: Measuring well-being.* OECD Publishing.

Orlik, W., Aleo, G., Kearns, T., Briody, J., Wray, J., Mahon, P., et al. (2022). Economic evaluation of CPD activities for healthcare professionals: A scoping review. *Medical Education.*

Ostir, G. V., Markides, K. S., Black, S. A., & Goodwin, J. S. (2000). Emotional well-being predicts subsequent functional independence and survival. *Journal of the American Geriatrics Society, 48*(5), 473–478.

Richards, M., & Huppert, F. A. (2011). Do positive children become positive adults? Evidence from a longitudinal birth cohort study. *The Journal of Positive Psychology, 6*(1), 75–87.

Rotenstein, L. S., Ramos, M. A., Torre, M., Segal, J. B., Peluso, M. J., Guille, C., et al. (2016). Prevalence of depression, depressive symptoms, and suicidal ideation among medical students: A systematic review and meta-analysis. *JAMA, 316*(21), 2214–2236.

Shah, M., Roggenkamp, M., Ferrer, L., Burger, V., & Brassil, K. J. (2021). Mental health and COVID-19: The psychological implications of a pandemic for nurses. *Clinical Journal of Oncology Nursing, 25*(1), 69–75.

Sibony, A. (2020). The UK COVID-19 response: A behavioral irony? *European Journal of Risk Regulation, 11*(2), 350–357.

Sriharan, A., West, K. J., Almost, J., & Hamza, A. (2021). Covid-19-related occupational burnout and moral distress among nurses: A rapid scoping review. *Nursing Leadership (Toronto, Ont.), 34*(1), 7–19.

Stone, A. A., Krueger, A. B., Stiglitz, J. E., Fitoussi, J. P., & Durand, M. (2018). Understanding subjective well-being. In *For good measure: Advancing research on well-being metrics beyond GDP* (pp. 163–201). OECD Publishing.

Thusini, S. (2020). Critical care nursing during the Covid-19 pandemic: A story of resilience. *British Journal of Nursing, 29*(21), 1232–1236.

United Nations Children's Fund. (2021). *Rapid review of global social protection responses to the Covid-19 pandemic Montenegro country brief*, New York.

Urquijo, L. G. (2021). The implementation of the European pillar of social rights (EPSR) in the post-pandemic era. *Romanian Journal of European Affairs, 21*(2), 85–94.

Van Hout, D., Hutchinson, P., Wanat, M., Pilbeam, C., Goossens, H., et al. (2022). The experience of European hospital-based health care workers on following infection prevention and control procedures and their well-being during the first wave of the COVID-19 pandemic. *PLoS One, 17*(2), e0245182.

Veenhoven, R. (1994). El estudio de la satisfacción con la vida. *Intervención Psicosocial, 3*, 87–116.

WHO. (2001). *The World Health Report 2001: Mental health: New understanding, new hope*. WHO.

WHO. (2016). *High-level commission on health employment and economic growth: Report of the expert group*. WHO.

WHO. (2022). *Mental health and COVID-19: Early evidence of the pandemic's impact: Scientific brief*. WHO.

Williams, W. C., Morelli, S. A., Ong, D. C., & Zaki, J. (2018). Interpersonal emotion regulation: Implications for affiliation, perceived support, relationships, and well-being. *Journal of Personality and Social Psychology, 115*(2), 224.

Xing, M. (2013). Molecular pathogenesis and mechanisms of thyroid cancer. *Nature Reviews Cancer, 13*(3), 184–199.

Manuel Lillo-Crespo is a Professor of the Department of Nursing, Faculty of Health Sciences, University of Alicante (Spain). He is a Vice-director at Vistahermosa HLA Hospital in Alicante. With experience in Team Leadership and Management of International Research Projects. Fellow of the Royal College of Surgeons in Ireland (RCSI) and Founder-Academic of the Nursing Academy at the Comunidad Valenciana. His areas of expertise are: Clinical and Healthcare Management and Administration, Nursing and Medical Professional Development, Healthcare/Clinical Anthropology (based on Qualitative Research Methodology and Mixed-Methods), and Educational Research and Innovation.

Chapter 10
The Well-being of Marginalized Migrants in Europe During the Covid-19 Epidemic: Evidence from France, Sweden, and the UK

Louise Dalingwater, Elisabeth Mangrio, Michael Strange, and Slobodan Zdravkovic

Abstract International guidance set forth recommendations to protect marginalized migrant populations during Covid-19 given the significant inequalities in terms of social and economic well-being reported in the literature. However, a cross-country study of three European countries with high rates of Covid-19 infections and deaths has shown that migrant well-being has significantly decreased since the outbreak of Covid-19 in Europe from March 2020 and that policy measures to help those marginalized populations have been insufficient. The conclusions on migrant well-being during Covid-19 draw on interviews with prominent civil society organizations in all three countries that work specifically on migrant health and welfare. All interviews were semi-structured and conducted between October and November 2020. The analysis mainly focuses on objective/material measures of well-being related to access to health care, information on prevention of infection, housing and exclusion by host population.

10.1 Introduction

Migration health and well-being has become a central pillar of EU health policy. Already in 2007, the Portuguese Presidency defined it as a key indicator of integration within host societies (Peiro & Benedict, 2010). Moreover, human rights treaties define the importance of equality so that everyone has the right to the "enjoyment of the highest attainable standard of physical and mental health" across all member

L. Dalingwater (✉)
Sorbonne Université, Paris, France
e-mail: louise.dalingwater@sorbonne-universite.fr

E. Mangrio · M. Strange · S. Zdravkovic
Malmö University, Malmö, Sweden

© The Author(s), under exclusive license to Springer Nature Switzerland AG 2022   177
L. Dalingwater et al. (eds.), *The Unequal Costs of Covid-19 on Well-being in Europe*,
Human Well-Being Research and Policy Making,
https://doi.org/10.1007/978-3-031-14425-7_10

states (OHCHR, 2002). However, in practice, migrants, especially the undocumented and asylum seekers have been found to have lower socio-economic status and reduced chances of achieving good health. At an international level, migrants' well-being has been a focus for the development of the OECD's well-being indicators. Such measures reveal that migrants suffer from greater poverty, have lower levels of income and wealth, and are more exposed to poorer housing and environmental conditions than non-migrants. They also found that migrants are less satisfied with their lives (OECD, 2017). International NGOs have confirmed that refugees, asylum seekers, and irregular migrant populations across Europe are more often than not living in poverty and destitution, which can explain poor health performance and lower levels of subjective well-being (Médécins du Monde, 2009; Médécins Sans Frontières, 2005).

More specifically the impact of Covid-19 on vulnerable migrants has been the focus of a number of empirical studies. However, the research is far from complete or comprehensive. Our study of the impact of Covid-19 focuses on three European countries, France, Sweden, and the UK, which all recorded high rates of Covid-19 infections and deaths. It draws on interviews with prominent civil society organizations in the three countries that work specifically on migrant health and welfare. All interviews were semi-structured and conducted between October and November 2020. The analysis mainly focuses on objective and material measures of well-being related to access to health care, information on prevention of infection, housing and discrimination by host populations. This chapter thus starts by presenting the conceptual framework we use to analyse migrant well-being, and considers general barriers to health and social care that migrants often face before presenting the empirical evidence on the three countries under study.

10.2   A Conceptual Framework to Analyse Migrant Well-being

When considering the well-being of vulnerable migrants in the context of the three European countries under study, it is particularly relevant to point to what Dluzewska (2016) has identified as the three most significant approaches to well-being in social sciences. The first is related to normative ideals (religious, cultural, and philosophical), the second to individual preferences and satisfaction, and the third to individual experiences. This paper will focus specifically on the third because it examines vulnerable migrants' experiences during Covid-19 and considers short- and long-term potential impacts on health outcomes. In addition, other important considerations within the literature on well-being, which are particularly relevant to our analysis of migrant well-being, are those identified in the Millennium Ecosystem Assessment which uses 5 main indicators to assess human well-being: health status, basic material wealth, social relations, security, and freedom of choice and action. Poverty within this framework is identified as the extremal deprivation of well-being (Carpenter et al., 2009; Dluzewska, 2016). These drivers of well-being are therefore particularly relevant to our cross-country study because they enable us to identify significant population welfare issues.

Hobfoll's Conservative of Resource Theory (1989) is also important to the study of migrant well-being. His theory explains that people are motivated by the need to retain, protect, and build resources to maintain well-being (material or subjective). However, since resources are not always distributed evenly, those with low economic status tend to be more vulnerable to the depletion of resources. Fisher (2019) uses Hobfoll's theory to develop a public well-being theory which depends on the objective nature of one's situation but also the subjective evaluation of that situation. Fisher argues that vulnerable migrants (and in his study more specifically migrant workers) experience lower well-being because they have low socio-economic status and are exposed to social discrimination.

Muoka and Hussier (2020) found that migration and precarious employment led to adverse health outcomes and diminished well-being. The results were obtained from a systematic review of peer-reviewed qualitative studies on migrants in precarious employment in the UK. In particular, musculoskeletal pain, exhaustion, anxiety, and depression resulted from precarious employment. Inequalities in health which can impact on overall well-being factors are related to a broad number of social determinants: barriers to access to health services but also poor living conditions and racial discrimination. The OECD's study on migrant health reported that poverty leads to the deterioration of migrant well-being in host societies in a number of ways: through poor housing, difficulties to access education, and inequitable distribution of income which can lead to marginalization and can more generally damage social cohesion (OECD, 2017). The report also underlines that good health is central to migrant well-being because it means migrants can work, earn more, and build broader social networks. However, there are a number of structural barriers for migrant populations to receive the health care and social provision they require.

10.3 Structural Barriers to Accessing Health and Social Care for Migrant Populations and the Impact on Well-being

Many young immigrants have been reported to have good health on arrival but their health advantages diminish over time (Brindis et al., 1995; Gfroerer & Tan, 2003). There are a number of explanations for the decline in health performance of migrants from developing countries over time including limitations on access to health services, working conditions, housing and other social conditions, adoption of poorer health behaviours and lifestyles in destination countries, barriers to health services, and neglecting one's own health owing to the priority to provide for families abroad (by sending money back home, for example). Moreover, the migratory process has been found to bring with it tensions which affect psychological health and well-being; owing to the decision to move itself and the implications of having to leave family behind (Carlisle, 2006). A joint WHO and IOM report found that stress-related conditions place a significant burden on migrant populations and thus considerable demands on the health systems of destination countries (WHO/IOM, 2010, p. 116). Hargreaves (2020) argues that refugees often find themselves excluded from national healthcare systems, face significant inequalities such as socio-cultural barriers, xenophobic attitudes from the general public but also healthcare professionals.

So a number of system- and patient-level barriers are apparent which are worth mentioning in more detail:

10.3.1 Barriers to Access to Health Services

These barriers can stem from a number of reasons, not limited to: lack of knowledge of publicly funded systems, barriers to access due to opening hours, distance, or cost, language barriers or cultural misunderstandings, and, lack of trust owing to one's legal status (Scheppers et al., 2006). A study on Sweden, which has been a significant receiving and hosting state for migrants, found that refugees' illegal status and lack of identity cards stopped them from using health services (MSF, 2005).

Structural barriers also include health literacy issues, which were clear from another study carried out in Sweden which found that most refugees had poor health literacy. This prevented them from accessing and understanding health information (Wångdahl et al., 2014). A similar study in the UK found that African migrant communities also had issues accessing health information and the lack of health literacy skills and language proficiency was an issue (Laverack, 2018).

10.3.2 Decline of Health Over Time

The decline in health is mainly owing to structural problems: housing problems, living in poor quality lodging, exploitative rents, crowded accommodation (Parrado et al., 2010). Indeed, evidence suggests that overcrowded, noisy, and insecure housing can have a serious impact on mental and physical health. Migrants may also be working in dangerous industries and hazardous jobs. The WHO Commission on Social Determinants of Health found that migrant workers were often concentrated in agricultural, food processing, construction, semi-skilled or unskilled manufacturing jobs, and low-wage service jobs. So low wage and hazardous working (exposure to chemicals, pesticides) can lead to a decline in health of migrants. Job precarity also adds to physical and mental health conditions particularly if wages are insufficient to support families. Migrants are also more likely to be exposed to work hazards (according to the WHO Commission).

It is important to note the complexity of migrant health interventions which can raise barriers to the provision of long-term health care. A Parisian doctor treating newly arrived migrants underlined the complexity of treating vulnerable migrants. The doctor reported that it was necessary to devote a whole morning to see five migrant patients, whereas standard consultations only took approximately 10 to 15 minutes. Doctors taking care of newly arrived migrants must mix medical diagnosis and social interviews. They will need to create a new health record for them because there may be no trace of the previous health history. They ask questions about the patient's migratory route, his or her accommodation, his or her diet, vaccinations, blood tests. Long and complex health interventions are thus required to make the correct diagnosis. In addition, time must be taken to establish trust with health practitioners. In some cases there is mistrust of Western medicine or medical practices.

10.3.3   Discriminatory Practices

While article 12 of the 1966 International Covenant on Economic, Social and Cultural rights (ICESCR) recognizes the rights of all human beings to enjoy the highest attainable standard of physical and mental health, in many European countries irregular migrants are not entitled to receive publicly funded healthcare free, with the exception of emergency care. Infectious diseases may be treated as an emergency. For asylum seekers in particular, the situation across European countries in terms of entitlements and access to services varies greatly (Norredam et al., 2006).

Where there are restrictive policies in place, health professionals across Europe may support such policies towards particular migrant groups. It is likely that views will vary amongst individuals and regionally, depending on levels of migration and/or perceived levels of health tourism. For example, a qualitative study in the UK exploring access to maternity information among recently arrived Somali women found that punitive attitudes and prejudiced views among health professionals led to reduced access to necessary services (Myfanwy & Davies, 2001). In the UK again, general practitioners (GPs) have in some cases been found to be reluctant to register asylum seekers and refugees and other new migrants because they may be highly mobile and are more difficult to follow-up for routine screening and vaccination (Hargreaves & Burnett, 2008). Exclusion can therefore result from this complicated and multi-layered organizational structure of health systems (Myfanwy & Davies, 2001; Papadopoulos et al., 2004; Priebe et al., 2011).

Trumer et al. (2010) identified significant disparities in Europe in terms of access to health care. They found that UK undocumented migrants, for example, have fewer rights to access to health care than in France but also the Netherlands, Spain, and Portugal. Availability of health care thus depends on European states' legislature. Insurance-based health systems such as France can give better access because the system enables them to differentiate between legal access and funding. Provision of health care also depends on the activity of NGOs working in migrant communities.

Medécins du Monde and Medecins sans Frontières are particularly active in France and the UK. In particular, when migrants are undocumented or illegal, health practitioners often find themselves faced with a predicament: break the migration law/financial regulations of the country by providing health care to the undocumented or violate human rights laws and public health norms by refusing treatment. In European countries, the denial of access to enter Europe and within this framework barriers to healthcare has been termed "Fortress Europe". Poor health is therefore related to how institutions deal with the undocumented and allow access to health provision. Health and well-being is dependent on the structural context, whether it be historical, social, political, or economic in which individuals find themselves and this significantly affects their agency (Isaacs et al., 2022).

As poverty is raised as an important issue, it is important to note that poverty in the UK has been found to be a result of the UK asylum process, whereby asylum seekers are entitled to only £39.63 (€44.01; 51.27 USD) a week (UK Government, 2020). Poverty means that refugees are unable to afford healthy food, pay the necessary travel to consult or access health services, and find meaningful employment. This is also the case in France and Sweden. Health risks developed during the asylum process can lead to reduced health outcomes over time. Long legal procedures and life pressures (the need to find a job, rent, etc.) lead to decreased health and well-being over time (Isaacs et al., 2022). Structural barriers thus prevent refugees and asylum seekers from accessing the necessary resources to lead a healthy life (Isaacs et al., 2022). Given that short-term factors can have a significant impact on health and well-being in the long term or exacerbate already existing social inequities, the empirical data collected in three European countries with different welfare traditions seems particularly relevant.

10.4 Empirical Study of Migrant Well-being During Covid-19

10.4.1 Background

A number of studies have emerged on the plight of vulnerable migrants during Covid-19 which show that they are at increased risk of infection because of substandard living conditions. Already existing literature has shown that migrant populations have been disproportionately affected by the Covid-19 crisis. For example, Hayward et al.'s (2021) systematic review of 3016 data sets in high-income countries, looking at hospitalizations, deaths, indirect health, and social effects among vulnerable migrants, found that there has been a disproportionate representation of migrants in reported Covid-19 deaths and an increased all-cause mortality in 2020. This might be explained by the fact that migrants are exposed to higher levels of risk factors and vulnerabilities owing to precarious occupations, overcrowded accommodation, legal-administrative barriers to health services, and other structural barriers limiting their well-being. Factors impacting on migrant health during Covid-19 thus mirror previously identified health risk factors (Nooria et al., 2021). In particular, low levels of language proficiency have meant that certain migrants have been excluded from the public health response (Nezafat Maldonado et al., 2020). Precarious occupations and difficult social situations have meant that vulnerable migrants have been excluded from Covid-19 population protection initiatives such as work from home, self-isolation, avoidance of public transport, and rapid testing (Hayward et al., 2021). Barriers to health services were also recognized in the literature review with thousands of migrants being reported to be excluded from health systems because of migration status, which meant exclusion from testing, treatment, and vaccine roll out. Potter et al. (2020) underline that migrants will often only seek access to health services for urgent treatment because of lack of trust, lack of knowledge of the health system, barriers to get registered, and general access. Dempster and Zimmer's (2020) study based on eight host countries, found that refugees are 60% more likely than host populations to be working in sectors which have been the most impacted by Covid-19 and notably accommodation and food services, manufacturing and retail. They also argue that the health and economic impacts of Covid are most likely to lead to greater loss of lives and more entrenched poverty among refugee populations. Refugees have had more difficulty accessing the labour market, claiming social safety nets and shielding themselves from disease.

Migrants also tend to be at the receiving end of the effects of economic recession: increased unemployment and rising xenophobia. Much of the discrimination reported during Covid-19 has been towards Chinese people owing to the emphasis, particularly at the beginning of the pandemic, on the geographical provenance of the disease (Alston et al., 2020; Croucher et al., 2020; Huo, 2020). Nevertheless, Meleady et al. (2021) found that there was also more widespread discrimination and blaming of ethnic minorities for spreading disease in areas with high numbers of Covid cases. This is because pandemics and the subsequent health and economic fallout may generate feelings of threat, uncertainty, and fear (Adam-Troian & Arciszewski, 2020; Van Bavel et al., 2020). The most vulnerable in society then become scape goats. Precise statistical information on undocumented migrants is not available but it is clear that from a number of empirical studies, discrimination and reduced access to health care, increased risk because of the inability to adhere to social distancing have placed vulnerable migrants at risk during Covid-19. While the literature is emerging, it is far from complete and exhaustive, so our research is an attempt to add to this emerging literature.

10.4.2   The Results of Our Research

Three countries were chosen to observe how Covid-19 affected vulnerable migrant populations, who were already suffering from a significant number of barriers to accessing health services and facing substandard living conditions, all of which contributed to lower levels of health and well-being. Much of the following analysis is on the undocumented. The focus on the undocumented is very important because to date there is little quantitative data in this area. The three countries were chosen both for pragmatic reasons—the background of co-authors with strong research bases in the three countries, but also to provide three quite contrasting situations. France, Sweden, and the UK have different social and economic traditions, which have an impact on the management of migrant issues. These three countries are also of interest because the death tolls per capita from Covid-19 were very high overall, especially in France and the UK, but similar in terms of deaths per capita (2558.67 per million population in the UK, France 2361.79, and Sweden 1815. 04 as of 24 April 2022).

The empirical evidence was collected between October and November 2020. The research draws on interviews with prominent civil society organizations in the three countries (3 France, 4 Sweden, 2 UK), working to improve migrant health and welfare. It shows how civil society groups have become facilitators to ensure that migrants have access to health and social care. The questions raised during the semi-structured interviews attempted to analyse the impact on migrant well-being: namely, access to health services, subsistence/poverty issues, and discrimination. These main factors were identified previously in the literature as having a significant impact on objective and subjective migrant well-being. The socio-economic conditions of migrants during Covid-19 were found to have worsened in the three countries under study during Covid-19, which raises significant concern as to the long-term impacts on migrant health and overall well-being.

10.4.2.1 France

The immigrant population living in France has grown from 4% to 10% of the population over the last century. This increase occurred in three major phases. In the 1920s, many of France's neighbours (Italians and Spaniards in particular) arrived to flee poverty and France needed workers to make up for the enormous loss of life due to the First World War. But afterwards, they returned or were sent back home, so that in 1946 immigrants represented only 5% of the population in France. In a second phase, their share increased relatively steadily in the post-war period until the early 1970s to reach 7%. Once again, France needed more workers during the *Trente Glorieuses*. Labour immigration then stabilized until the end of the 1990s. But from the 2000s onwards, a third wave occurred and immigrants represented 10.3% of the population in 2021.

In 2020, despite a decrease in migratory movements towards Europe, to the order of 29% compared to 2018, France experienced a sharp increase in asylum applications. In 2018, France registered a record 123,000 asylum applications, an increase of 22% compared to the previous year when asylum applications were already high. At the same time, the number of asylum applications fell by 10% in the rest of Europe. This was particularly evident in Italy (58%), Hungary (80%), Austria (46%), and Germany (17%) (Assemblée Nationale, 2020). France thus finds itself in a unique situation with regard to its European partners due to two phenomena:

1. A significant intake of migrants is owing to secondary migratory movements from other European countries. On average, 30% of asylum seekers in France have already lodged an application in another EU Member State and are not, according to European law, France's responsibility (the "dublined");
2. It receives a large proportion of asylum applications from nationals of countries that France considers to be safe.

The significant increase in asylum applications in France has consequences for the cost of the allowance received by applicants and the financing of accommodation structures, leading each year, as the Court of Auditors noted last spring, to an overstretched system. No satisfactory political solution has yet been found at national or European level.

Another key challenge is that interventions to deal with migratory pressures are very much devolved to the local level in France. Associations are the main actors providing support to newly arrived migrants at that level. Some of these associations are financed by the *Fonds d'Action Social (FAS)* which is a national agency with regional offices and through the municipalities. Policies do not directly target migrants but rather neighbourhoods and vulnerable persons. There is however mention of immigration populations and integration issues in central state and local authority contracts (Geddes & Scholten, 2016). However, there are marked differences between localities in terms of the health and social care provided to vulnerable migrants as a number of studies have shown (Garbaye, 2005). The interviews were carried out in three areas where there is significant pressure and under-capacity: Paris, Calais, and the Grande Synthe[1] regions.

Access to Health Care

Out of the three countries, theoretically France appears to have the best access to both emergency and general health services. The undocumented, asylum seekers, refugees, or holders of a residence permit are entitled to medical assistance on the same basis as French nationals. Migrants regardless of their status can benefit from universal cover either through the *Aide médicale d'État (AME)* or the *Couverture maladie universelle complémentaire (CMU-C)*. Both systems allow all migrants irrespective of their status to claim state medical aid. Doctors in France cannot refuse to treat patients even though refusals have been reported. However, both require migrants to prove that they have been in France for at least three months. Newly arrived migrants can receive health cover through health care access centres (*Permanences d'accès aux soins de santé* (PASS)). These are health centres located in public hospitals and intended for people without any health cover.

---

[1] Grande Synthe is in the North of France just outside Dunkirk.

However, in practice, there are a number of barriers to accessing health care for vulnerable migrants in France. Moreover, the French state has failed to implement adjustments to structures since the beginning of the Covid-19 pandemic in order to increase the provision of healthcare for migrants and overcome some of the barriers to providing healthcare to vulnerable people. Associations working with migrants, and notably *Medecins sans frontières* and *Medecins du monde* did however intervene on site to provide extra health services during the Covid-19 pandemic. However, barriers to health services are still significant. Associations working in the field believe that structures need to be more flexible and adapted to the reality of this population.

Even if the migrants technically have access to health services, in practice there are many obstacles which migrants have faced to access healthcare during Covid-19 which confirm the structural difficulties raised in the literature. First of all, access to information and health services is a problem. According to Doctors of the World France (DOWF), the structures are also not adapted to the vulnerable migrant population:

> The problems with exiled people is that [] they are in transit, they travel a lot from one place to another in the Paris region, the north, Belgium, etc. and that means that we, for example, operate on a mobile basis, we intervene directly in the places where people live and on several occasions we have asked the PASS to operate on a mobile basis and to adapt to the needs of population. (DOW France, Calais and Grande Synthe)

The issue of language problems was also raised in the interviews with very few interpreters in rare languages like Farci or Tashto being available to assist the migrants. The other issue was the inability for migrants to purchase medication once they have left the hospital or medical centre. Indeed, while some drugs are free of charge, the most recent ones to treat Covid-19 are quite costly.

While migrants living in crowded accommodation were at significant risk from contracting Covid-19, the most excluded and vulnerable living on the streets were considered not to be as exposed to the virus:

> As the director of the Calais hospital said at a recent meeting, he considers that the migrant population is not a population at risk because they are young and because of their way of life, of surviving, they live outside, practically the only shelters they have are tents or tarpaulins, and these conditions are less likely to spread the virus. (Auberge des migrants).

But it was also noted that it is very difficult to test this population for infection and so the information on the risk of contracting Covid-19 for this population on the street was not clearly established:

> What I would add is that it is possible that there were a lot of people who had flu-like symptoms perhaps from Covid but who did not consult/get tested. We were at the end of the winter when the government started to take serious measures against the pandemic and there were a lot of people among them who had rhino pharyngitis, coughs etc. and so it is also possible that these people were ill, not too seriously, but that they did not get tested. There were perhaps many more positive cases than one might think. (Auberge des migrants)

What was also clear from the interviews was that health was unfortunately not a priority. As one volunteer in the Calais region described, there were often other priorities:

> You have to understand that the people who are in Calais are there because they want to go to Great Britain and their energy, their attention is focused on this question of the crossing and not necessarily even sometimes on their sorry condition. That is to say that when we speak with them sometimes they say yes, it's true, it's hard but anyway, maybe tomorrow I'll be gone or the day after tomorrow, so they're also in that state of mind that makes them tolerate difficult conditions of survival. The same goes for the virus. Maybe there were people who had a lot of symptoms, pulmonary or, of the cold type, headache but who did not necessarily get tested. (Auberge des migrants)

The lack of priority migrants give to personal health is cause for concern, as one volunteer explained:

> There are even people who are very sick but they are not going to go to the hospital for treatment because they don't want to be hospitalized for weeks and months in France. (Auberge des migrants).

The migrants are reluctant to go to hospital because it may prevent them from crossing the channel to reach the UK. The volunteer from DOWF also underlined very much the same issue, that it was difficult to raise awareness because Covid-19 was very much a secondary issue for the migrants:

> It was a secondary problem, so we were not able to have much impact on the information we passed on because for them the priority was to find food, to eat, to have shelter for the night, and Covid was something very far removed for them. [] They told us they thought it was a Western disease, it was a disease that didn't concern them. (DOW France)

Subsistence Issues

Indeed, vulnerable migrants in Europe, as we have seen in the literature, are particularly vulnerable to deterioration in health and well-being owing to severe levels of poverty. The interviews revealed that Covid-19 exacerbated the situation for many of them. The housing problem for migrants is not a new issue in France, especially in densely populated cities such as Paris. Policy measures initiated at national level and implemented at the local level proved to be inadequate to meet the needs of the populations concerned, especially in the Paris region or in complex situations like those in Calais where migrants arrive in order to attempt to travel across to Britain.

The French state did increase funding to house the homeless during lockdown. It is worth noting that an ever increasing number of marginalized migrants are among the homeless. 178,800 extra shelter spots in France for homeless people (including asylum seekers) were provided from March to May 2020. According to official reports, 3600 places in centres were opened from March 2020 across France to provide shelter for the homeless suffering from Covid-19 but who do not require hospitalization. Provision of basic necessities for homeless people without any other resources was increased. Indeed, from April 2020, service vouchers (7 euros per day/person) were distributed for more than 130,000 people (including nearly 14,000 in overseas France), which could be used in 250,000 stores throughout France.

By law, the state has an obligation to provide shelter and food for these populations. However, it is often the case that there is a lack of capacity. The OFII (housing office) is often not able to provide accommodation because they receive too many requests and accommodation is too crowded. In which case, they give an additional allowance of 200 euros per month. However, this allowance does not even cover 4 nights' accommodation in Paris or in other key agglomerations either.

According to a social worker at the association Aurore, in Paris, despite the provision of extra housing after the first lockdown in March 2020, the situation has worsened in terms of providing accommodation for marginalized migrants who come to their day centre for assistance and for the possibility of being transferred to suitable accommodation. The association noted that while the government created more places, this was not at all evident at the grassroots level:

> The vast majority of them don't have any accommodation. What they are looking for really when they come here is to leave for a transfer to a centre where they are provided accommodation[2] and the problem is that since the beginning of lockdown, the places have been drastically reduced (. . .) the problem is that in the evening these men have to go back to makeshift camps, at Porte d'Aubervilliers for example, although now the camps have shifted further out of Paris to Saint Denis, and in the evening they have nothing, they sleep as best they can.

> Lockdown happened and everything stopped. For two months there was no possibility of transfer for asylum seekers to the accommodation centres, many of these people experienced the lockdown as best they could, sleeping on trains, in stations and these transfers only resumed again during the month of May, but we only have 24 places per week instead of the usual 90, so that means we have lost 66 places. (Aurore, Paris)

The volunteer at Aurore underlined that the accommodation that was provided was sometimes inadequate:

> A man [who came to the day centre] was offered a place to sleep at a gym, a gym where social distancing was not respected. He said to me "the Covid measures are not put in place, what's the point". It was not the right place to be during lockdown . . . . (Aurore, Paris)

---

[2] These centres provide accommodation for migrants occupying the illegal camps in north-east Paris who have been directed via the regular round ups or referred to by one of the two day centres run by the regional prefecture. During their stay, which lasts on average 10 days, migrants can benefit from health, social, and administrative support before registering their asylum application with the *Guichet Unique pour Demande d'Asile (GUDA)*, located close to the CAES. Depending on their administrative situation, migrants are then redirected to structures adapted to their situation in Ile-de-France (Paris region), while their asylum application is being processed. On 1 January 2020, the national reception system had around 43,600 authorized places in reception centres for asylum seekers (CADA). The accommodation is mainly located in Ile-de-France, Auvergne-Rhône, and Grand Est. However, the largest number of new centres have been created in the Pays de la Loire, Brittany, New Aquitaine, and Occitania regions. The main operator is ADOMA and then COALLIA, FTDA, Forum réfugiés-Cosi. In recent years, the SOS group and France Horizon have developed an important network.

In Calais, the Auberge des migrants volunteer was also critical of the interventions to attempt to house the migrants during lockdown:

> A certain number of people did leave to stay in the accommodation but they came back quickly because the material conditions, among other things, were considered not to be good. And besides, it's quite paradoxical because the migrants were put in these rooms, notably in an old Formula 1 hotel in Boulogne sur Mer and they were three or four to a room and therefore they found themselves in a context which was perhaps more likely to spread the virus than in their camps and under their tents. (Auberge des migrants).

The housing crisis has thus exacerbated the situation for migrants and their exposure to Covid-19 and vulnerable migrants have seen a deterioration in living conditions during Covid-19 in France. According to *Médécins sans Frontières* (MSF), one in two marginalized persons (90% marginalized migrants) tested positive for Covid-19. Conducted between 23 June and 2 July, the MSF study revealed large disparities according to the types of sites where people were tested. In ten of the accommodation centres, the positivity rate reached 50.5%, compared with 27.8% in the food distribution sites and 88.7% in the two migrant worker hostels. MSF explained that the main reason for such disparities was owing to unsuitable shelter which creates clusters. For example, in gymnasiums where homeless migrants were housed during lockdown and migrant worker hostels, the sanitary conditions did not meet Covid-19 safety standards. This resulted in a large majority of workers testing positive to coronavirus.

A DOWF volunteer also underlined that conditions had deteriorated for the migrants since the outbreak of Covid-19. First, she mentioned that the extra housing and initiatives were only in place during the three months of lockdown and since then all these extra initiatives to take care of vulnerable persons such as migrants have been disbanded:

> Living conditions are extremely difficult in the camps and it's true that during lockdown everything was that bit worse. During lockdown, the State put in place access to water, access to showers and so on in the Grande Synthe area, and at the end of lockdown everything was removed, so it was a fairly short period. However, the situation is still as complex as ever before in the Grande Synthe area, there is one water point, 6 toilets for 400 people and no access to showers. (DOW France).

In the Calais and Grande Synthe regions, access to food and other basic necessities became that much harder after March 2020:

> The lockdown has worsened the situation of the exiles since a certain number of associations have either stopped altogether or have reduced their activities. I am thinking of the Catholic Relief Service (Secours Catholique), which has a daytime reception, it has closed, whereas it used to welcome 100, 150 people for different things, for rest, a bit of leisure, etc. They closed down and there is the English Refugee Community Kitchen, which stopped altogether because the volunteers, who were mainly British, were afraid of not being able to get back to go to Great Britain and so they went back at the beginning of lockdown. So there was rather a deterioration of migrants' lives during this period. (Auberge des migrants)

On a positive note, the volunteer at the Paris day centre noted that there was a certain degree of solidarity and donations from people, food banks, and restaurant owners who made meals for the migrants. Moreover, it would seem these extreme conditions of lack of access to food were specifically a problem during the first lockdown. Nevertheless, the conditions more generally of worsening poverty and living conditions can be said to have a significant impact on migrant health and well-being in France.

Discrimination

Heightened discrimination was also an issue raised in the interviews. The volunteer at the Paris day centre underlined how the necessity to have a certificate and a place of residence to self-isolate during the first lockdown led to the discrimination of the migrant homeless:

> If they wandered around on the street, they had to have a certificate.[3] This was the most difficult thing to make people understand because they were actually on the street. How can you be in lockdown when you sleep here and there, where you can, that was the most difficult thing for them and many of them were fined by the police. This is one of the big problems, already there is the language problem for them, the police speak French, not necessarily English, the police did not understand and did not have time to understand the situation of these gentlemen, and in fact they were just on the street and they were still being punished for it. (Aurore, Paris)

A volunteer in Calais also underlined how the Covid-19 restrictions have served as an excuse to harden the action against illegals:

> The hardening of the government's policy over the last two months is evident because there has been an increase in the number of evacuations, there has been a reduction in the services that the state should provide to the exiles so as to discourage them from staying in Calais. (Auberge des migrants)

More generally, a volunteer in Calais underlined how the discrimination of the French state towards this population actually represented a violation of human rights:

> We criticise the government's policy in Calais publicly whenever we can, not only from a humanitarian point of view, it's a policy that is inhumane, that puts people in difficult conditions of survival, but it's also a policy that is very costly, that is ineffective and that is contrary to human rights on so many levels and in any case contrary to the values of our country. (Auberge des migrants)

The same volunteer underlined that the possibility to carry out identity checks in the street in France, means that the chances of being picked up by the police are greater and these checks have increased since the beginning of the pandemic:

> In Great Britain, you don't have to show your identity card in the street, in France you have to, so in France migrants are subject to identity checks quite often and this obviously increases their chances of being arrested, put in a detention centre and deported. In Great

---

[3] During lockdown in France, it was only permitted to leave one's house for one hour per day and it was necessary to be in possession of a signed statement which indicated the time you left your house.

Britain, there are checks in shops, there are checks in workshops, especially inspections following denunciation, but there are not many of them and someone who is illegal can manage to survive there for several years and send money back home to his family without necessarily being arrested and deported. (Auberge des migrants)

A DOWF volunteer mentioned that the police would use identity checks as an excuse to request undocumented migrants using the buses to step down and this often led to the migrants failing to gain access to health or social care services.

The volunteers were also aware of an upsurge in discrimination since the outbreak of Covid-19, both in the streets and on social media:

As a result, on the social networks, we have of course seen comments such as "yes migrants are sheltered, housed, fed, etc., whereas we homeless people don't get any shelter and food (…)"

It always come from the same sources of the extreme right-wing parties and then a part of public opinion which expresses itself on social networks and which is anti-migrant for the wrong reasons or very wrong reasons. That is to say, it can go from the simple expression of discomfort and it is true that in Calais the presence of migrants with no accommodation can sometimes cause problems, and this goes from the simple expression of discomfort to downright racist comments. (Auberge des migrants)

Discrimination owing to the difficulties that migrants have to social distance, wear facial coverings was also a significant problem and the migrants were blamed for spreading the disease:

There are a lot of observations on the fact that social distancing was not respected by migrants in the queues. In the food distribution by La Vie Active, the government organisation and ours, it is always difficult to respect the rules of distancing. Not all migrants have masks. The distribution of masks in France was late and it was even later for migrants, so it was only from July, August that there was some distribution made by La Vie Active, notably of masks to migrants, but never enough. (…) They can't necessarily wash their hands or change their clothes. It's obvious in their living conditions that it's very difficult to respect hygiene recommendations. We've seen it and many people have seen it and some have denounced it. (Auberge des migrants)

10.4.2.2 Sweden

People on the move, i.e., migration, is not new instead this is something that has been ongoing over the years. In Sweden, different trends have been observed during the last decade, from emigration at the end of nineteenth century and during the first part of the twentieth century, to immigration (Asyl, 2022). Some of the reasons for immigrating to Sweden have been labour, poverty, reunification, and war classified as voluntary or forced migration. During the last decade, most people coming to Sweden came from regions and countries with war. The majority applied for asylum on refuge grounds. The number of asylum application in 2015 was 162,877 including 51,338 coming from Syria. In 2016, Sweden changed the Reception of Asylum Seekers Act (LMA) and established a new temporary law resulting in temporary residence permits for approved asylum applications. These changes switched the reception from being very generous to restrictive (a.a.). The Swedish population consists today, at end of 2021, of 10,452,326 people coming from many parts of the world (SCB). The number of people being born outside the country was 2,090,503 at the end of last year which was approximately 20% of the population.

Out of the three countries, Sweden is usually identified as the most generous in terms of social welfare. It has an international reputation as a country which respects human rights and migrant rights to legal and welfare systems. During 2015, Sweden received a high influx of refugees coming mostly from Syria and Iraq. Around 160,000 refugees were registered as asylum seekers in Sweden that year. Due to the high reception of refugees, some restrictions in the law were implemented. More precisely, restrictions yielded limitation on permanent permissions to stay. Temporary permissions to stay have since then been more common. Furthermore, restrictions also included the right for the refugees already given resident permits to reunite with their family members being left in the country of origin.

Healthcare Access

All migrants in Sweden, including those with refugee status, undocumented and newly arrived refugees have the right to healthcare that cannot be deferred, which includes emergency physical and dental care, maternal care, abortion as well as healthcare connected to infectious diseases. In practice, this means that all healthcare that is required and that cannot be postponed is included (Sveriges, 2022).

However, even if Sweden has a generous healthcare system for migrants regardless of status, there have been some challenges in relation to migrants accessing healthcare. Large surveys conducted during the last years in the south part of Sweden have revealed that migrants have unmet healthcare needs. When asking newly arrived refugees if they had needed healthcare during the last 3 months but did not seek care, around 70% answered yes to that. The most frequent reason mentioned were cost and language difficulties. They also expressed a dissatisfaction with delays in waiting for appointments or waiting for referrals and others as well as they were expecting better follow-up care in regard to diabetes care, for example (Mangrio, 2018).

In the interviews carried out with civic communicators working closely with migrants and their healthcare in Sweden, the communicators expressed lack of clarity, on whether EU migrants were covered by universal health care. The understanding of the migrants' access to health care differed through the different regions in the country. EU migrants, which often mean Romani people, fall outside free health care cover.

> EU migrants fall outside of the covering health care system, since they have often been in Sweden more than 3 months as undocumented (DOW, Sweden)

Another challenge in regard to healthcare access during the pandemic has, according to interviewed civic communicators, been with the digital tools that are needed in order to get in contact with healthcare settings or book appointments, or for Covid testing. Civic society has warned that migrants groups in Sweden have had difficulties accessing healthcare when it has become dependent upon digital technology.

> The digitalization of the health care exclude groups in society. To not be able to enter a health care clinic, but being forced to call instead, make the access to care worse for this group. The automatic information in the health care phone lines is mainly adapted to Swedish and English people with personal numbers (Red Cross, Stockholm).

An additional observed challenge was communicating information about Covid-19 in translated versions, which was done by the Public Health Agency including films in different languages. The civic and health communicators were commissioned by the Public Health agency to work to disseminate information and they met refugees on a daily basis, during their classes within the establishment process and have engaged in answering questions that the newly arrived had around this subject. They also continuously worked on updating and disseminating new information from the public health agency. Further on, the transcultural centre in Stockholm also played a central role in informing migrant populations of Covid-19 and its preventative measures. On a daily basis, they have staffed a helpline where migrants have been able to seek information in their mother tongue.

Subsistence Issues

Housing and expenses for living are covered for all migrants that have received residence permits. These expenses are, however, covered only for migrants actively participating in the introduction programme given for migrants during their first 2 years in Sweden. Asylum seekers are, on the other hand, encouraged to support themselves and, if not possible, they have the right to receive some limited economic reimbursement.

In spite of getting economic support from the government regarding housing and food coverage, there is a shortage of housing facilities as well as difficulties finding apartments for migrants in Sweden. This is mainly due to apartment owners requiring migrants to show proof of employment which for the majority of the migrants is impossible as they are at the beginning of their stay in Sweden and as such are unemployed. Another challenge has been that the places that they manage to rent, often through contacts, are crowded and insecure. During the pandemic this matter has been highlighted since this matter has been even more acknowledged since crowded living increases the risk of Covid-19.

During an interview a worker from the Red Cross said:

> People are already living in vulnerable situations and have been more prone to vulnerability during the pandemic. The ones that suffer from no rights to support from the social welfare, have now been dependent on the civil society for support. A support, that the civil society, already before the pandemic, had a hard time to deliver (Red Cross).

Meeting places for migrants have also been closed down, due to restrictions on social contacts, which means a decline in the support/protection for these people that already are in higher needs of these places.

"Meeting places such as coffee places for migrants to socialize have been closed down, due to restrictions and these migrants suffer more due to their already vulnerable situation socially" (Red Cross Stockholm).

Discrimination

Discrimination towards migrants is something that is happening, it happened before the pandemic and has continued to be a threat to migrants well-being in Swedish society during the pandemic. A nurse at the Rosengrenska clinic said:

> When you are undocumented, you are already stigmatized and it is difficult to sink even further down that what they already are. This is since they live here illegally and unwanted because of their juridical status (Rosengrenska clinic).

She also said that they this was despite the virus having entered Sweden through rich Swedish holidaymakers coming home from the Alps and not through the refugees.

She then went on to explain:

> We have noticed that Covid-19 has made the social classes in society more evident and the rich people could work more from home and we have seen some... suffer more from Covid-19 due to their profession. This has been related more to which profession/work you hold than a lack of information or protection (Rosengrenska clinic).

Another matter of concern is the association between crowded living and the higher risk of catching Covid-19 and this knowledge could worsen the assumption that is built around migrants and risk from contracting Covid-19. The nurse at Rosengrenska also said:

> It could be that we assume that all migrants live in crowded conditions and therefore we have a stigmatized view on the migrants because of that (Rosengrenska clinic).

10.4.2.3   UK

The United Kingdom's migration history is marked by its role as a colonial power from the eighteenth through to the twentieth centuries, and in many ways that continues to the present through its continuing neocolonial role as an epicentre of major financial power and resource ownership that crosses the globe. In addition, the UK has been militarily active in key conflict zones. As a result, the UK sits at the centre of numerous migration routes, with both mass historical emigration to its former colonies, and as a country of immigration when those territories became independent. The UK is today noted for its self-proclaimed "hostile" immigration policies, and yet remains a highly attractive location for many persons from Africa and South East Asia. The primary reason for this is that several UK cities have large communities recently descended from those regions such that it is easier for newly arrived migrants from Africa and South East Asia to find work and social contacts than in many other wealthy countries. In particular, migrants residing in countries often perceived as having much more welcoming policies nevertheless find it hard to get work and, instead, choose to try and reach the UK.

The UK is a case in point whereby access to healthcare for the undocumented has become increasingly difficult as a result of harsh immigration policies. Health care is provided in the UK according to residency which included the undocumented until 2003. However, a law passed by the House of Lords changed the terminology to lawful residence and thus excluded undocumented migrants from access to health care. Health care has therefore been denied through the continued instrumentalization of immigration policy (Vernon, 2012). Indeed, in 2012, the home office in the UK implemented the hostile environment policy which was a set of administrative and legal measures intended to make life for the undocumented unbearably difficult. Employees in housing departments, schools, and hospitals with the specific title of "overseas payment officers" were thus employed in the UK to denounce illegal immigrants when they came to seek health or social care services. In one West Middlesex Hospital, a direct line between the hospital and immigration services was connected in 2008 and ward clerks were requested to report any patients who they suspected were not lawful residents to the overseas payment officers. The role of the latter was, namely, to charge patients rather than denounce them to immigration authorities, although the officer could fax queries to immigration authorities to check status, which could be seen to be indirect denunciation. In either case, it has strongly deterred those lacking permanent residency from seeking health care.

The UK's Home Office, that has central responsibility for asylum applications, thus operates a highly complex migration management system openly designed to undermine the living conditions and rights of asylum seekers, within a network that shares private data on such individuals across all spheres (i.e. policing, health, social services, education) where they might interact with the state, whilst outsourcing many of its responsibilities to private contractors (e.g. transportation, and detention facilities) and public workers legally obliged to help police migration laws (e.g. doctors, university staff) as well as private landlords required to restrict housing access.

Complex institutional hostility runs parallel with a practice of infamously slow processing rates for asylum applications, meaning individuals are left in limbo for extended periods, often at the mercy of predatory solicitors doing little to support their applications, whilst the UK government also bans asylum seekers from legal access to the labour market. The effect is that asylum seekers can often stay in the UK for much longer periods than compared to other European states, due to the slow processing of their cases, but in so doing are heavily marginalized. Lacking formal access to national social security benefits, families and individuals awaiting processing are often subject to "No Recourse to Public Funds" (NRPF) conditions, such that their access to housing and living costs is dependent upon the varying and often unreliable provision of services at the local municipal level, as well as ad hoc support from civil society or personal contacts.

Access to Health Services

In general, asylum seekers in the UK, including those refused permission to stay, should always receive medical treatment that is classed as "urgent" regardless of their ability to pay, but this means that they may still be billed at a later date, and cannot get treatment for conditions classed as "non-urgent" but nevertheless remain life-threatening (e.g. for cancer, or heart conditions) unless they can pay the prohibitively high costs. Evaluation of what constitutes an "urgent" condition rests on health practitioners, who by being required to ask after a patient's residency status, and to report irregular migrants to the Home Office, are brought directly into the migration policing system at the expense of their role as health providers. In all four nations of the UK, refugees and asylum seekers with an active application or appeal are entitled to free NHS care at the point of use.

Overseas visitors were allowed access to testing for coronavirus, as well as treatment. And, of most importance particularly for irregular migrants, no immigration checks are required for patients receiving only testing or treatment for coronavirus. However, according to Doctors of the World and the Institute of Race Relations, the effectiveness of this exception driven by Covid-19 has been greatly undermined in two ways. First, the UK government has been slow to communicate the exception to health practitioners, and information to migrants remains poor and often overly technical given language difficulties. Second, it is not always clear when the exceptions apply given that individuals may have multiple health conditions requiring treatment, and that could both lead to them being charged a fee, as well as having their information passed onto the UK's Home Office and the police, exposing them to deportation.

In an interview, an activist described the main issue as being a lack of trust due to past incidences of official initiatives presented as helping migrants being used as a cover to catch and detain those individuals for deportation:

> The government didn't do. . .an information campaign in all languages saying, "You can get this for free". So again it was down to the community groups to tell people but they themselves said "Well, we are not sure if we should because we don't know. . .whether people are then going to get picked up". So, this distrust is so profound and quite rightly. (IRR)

Due to many doctors' surgeries closing down during the lockdown, and providing restricted services afterwards, there has been an over-reliance on online services that often exclude vulnerable groups. According to DoW UK the situation meant *highly technologically literate people who just didn't have the technology and the resources to. . .make phone calls and to get online*. Often marginalized migrants lack their own phone, making it very difficult for them to book health care appointments, but also be contacted by GPs. In addition, whereas at the start of the pandemic the UK government decided to release some migrants from immigration detention for public health reasons, those individuals lost access to their usual source of healthcare and, at the same time, had difficulty contacting the GP surgeries within the communities where they were moved (DoW UK).

The lack of sufficient information clarifying what access asylum seekers and irregular migrants had to Covid-19 testing, mentioned above, put those individuals in an impossible situation where the positive news of not having the virus might risk them being charged for a lesser condition not exempted from fees, or being reported to the Home Office. An interview stated:

> It's impossible for a patient to make a decision about whether to go forward to services or what the risks for them are so it just means that they postpone it. . .until they become really desperate. Which is obviously a disaster for public health. (DoW UK)

Subsistence Issues

Asylum seekers awaiting a decision from the UK's Home Office are granted an allowance of only £5.39 a day per person (approximately 6 euros), provided usually in the form of vouchers or on a pre-paid card to be used at designated vendors. With no legal right to work whilst their cases are being processed, this automatically places asylum seekers in a state of abject poverty unless they have access to other means of income, which few do. During that period, the Home Office provides accommodation, but often only within extremely overcrowded facilities. Once an asylum claim has been approved, the Home Office no longer provides accommodation or financial support. Where then classed as a "refugee", the housing of those individuals falls under the responsibility of the local authority. The bureaucratic transition between being an "asylum seeker" to a "refugee" is rarely seamless, with delays exposing refugees to a high risk of being made homeless.

Living in a precarious situation means marginalized migrants were already particularly vulnerable, and where that precarity is strongest in the UK, the situation with Covid-19 has created a vicious circle. One health activist stated:

> People, as their lives are becoming more difficult. . .as their financial resources are drying up, as they can't buy soap and face masks and phone credit and can't speak to people and access to food is becoming harder and people. . . . accessing health care services is becoming further and further away from reality. (DoW UK)

One success of the UK response, noted in the interviews, was that at the start of the pandemic the national government demanded that local authorities put all homeless persons, including migrants, into hotels. In addition, there was also a temporary pause on all evictions from asylum accommodation, so that those with refused asylum claims could avoid being homeless during the lockdown in the Spring. At the same time, though, living conditions within the asylum accommodation system remained overcrowded, particularly for single men often forced to share a bed, and non-relatives having to share rooms, often without access to essential sanitation, like soap and face masks.

Furthermore, the policy to accommodate all homeless persons quickly led to more overcrowding. The national government also decided, at the height of the lockdown in Spring 2020, through its private contractors, so as to minimize the amount of journeys its staff would need to make to visit asylum seeker accommodation sites, to move approximately 300 individuals in Glasgow out of flats into mass accommodation units where individuals were suddenly forced to share transport and then rooms with complete strangers despite being urged to social distance, creating significant fear (Interview IRR).

The poor conditions in which many asylum seekers are forced to live, which worsened for some during the pandemic, were criticized by a civil society representative as follows:

> What is the point in offering them a test when you have created conditions for them to get Covid? And contained them in these circumstances. (IRR)

The UK government continued to restrict asylum seekers' accommodation, preventing them from legally renting rooms, as well as maintaining the criminalization of their seeking paid employment. Where either would have helped give them a better chance to self-protect from Covid-19, the failure to improve living conditions stands out as an omission to control the spread of the virus.

Discrimination

Whilst the UK government claims to be able to directly challenge false narratives that threaten society's well-being, having established a Counter Disinformation Cell led by the Department for Digital, Culture, Media and Sport, this largely focuses on whatever the government decides is a "false" on social media. In practice, although the "hostile society" mantra is no longer an official policy, the logic remains pervasive such that prominent Members of Parliament (MPs), including those in government positions, have frequently been accused of stigmatizing migrants.

In the context of Covid-19, the issue of anti-stigmatization of migrants in the UK has been absorbed within the much more prominent issue of anti-stigmatization of minority and vulnerable groups in general due to the actions of several MPs in blaming black and ethnic minorities for the gross disparities between Covid-19 infection rates amongst their communities compared to the wider population, whilst refusing to acknowledge evidence of structural racism as the key factor explaining such disparities.

According to DoW, in contrast to the stigmatization often pushed by the UK government, it has been civil society which has been leading anti-stigmatization efforts in the UK, to do "campaigning and media work on what the asylum system is, why we offer asylum, why accommodation is important and also why inappropriate accommodation is not okay". That also includes civil society campaigns to portray more positive stories on asylum seekers. That refers to a general anti-stigmatization campaign regarding migrants, rather than specific to Covid-19.

10.5 Conclusion

This chapter has sought to highlight the significant barriers which migrants face across Europe in accessing essential health care and accommodation. It also highlights discriminatory practices which represent both physical and psychological constraints to ensuring migrant health and well-being. The empirical evidence has shone light on the factors which have led to a deterioration in migrant well-being during the Covid-19 pandemic. Vulnerable migrants are clearly at risk because of pre-existing structural barriers to ensuring a minimum standard of living. It is evident that barriers to health care that existed before the pandemic are even more evident now. The policies that are currently being developed must therefore take into consideration how Covid-19 has further exacerbated both the physical and mental health of migrants. A more holistic approach to ensuring the future well-being and general social integration of migrants into society is necessary. In addition, as the pandemic has shown, failure to ensure all segments of the population—regardless of citizenship status—have access to quality healthcare undermines public health overall. There is a need to ensure that the lessons of Covid—where inequities and weaknesses in healthcare have been made grossly visible—are not now lost as we seek to make our world more resilient to future pandemics.

Acknowledgements Auberge des migrants, Calais, France
Aurore, Paris, France.
County government, Malmö.
Doctors of the World, UK.
Doctors of the World, Sweden,
Institute for Race Relations, UK.
Médecins du Monde, Calais and Grande Synthe.
Milena Milosavljevic, Malmö University.
Red Cross, Stockholm.
Rosengrenska, Health care clinic, Gothenburg.

References

Adam-Troian, J., & Arciszewski, T. (2020). Absolutist words from search volume data predict state-level suicide rates in the United States. *Clinical Psychological Science, 8*(4), 788–793. https://doi.org/10.1177/2167702620916925
Alston, L., Meleady, R., & Seger, C. R. (2020). Can past intergroup contact shape support for policies in a pandemic? Processes predicting endorsement of discriminatory Chinese restrictions during the COVID-19 crisis. *Group Processes & Intergroup Relations*. Advanced Online Publication. https://doi.org/10.1177/1368430220959710
Assemblée nationale. (2020). N° 2577 Assemblée nationale Constitution du octobre 1958.
Asyl. (2022). Migrationsverket. https://www.migrationsverket.se/Om-Migrationsverket/Statistik/Asyl.html. Accessed 13 Sept 2022
Brindis, C., Wolfe, A. L., McCarter, V., Ball, S., & Starbuck-Morales, S. (1995). The associations between immigrant status and risk-behavior patterns in Latino adolescents. *Journal of Adolescent Health, 17*, 99–105.

Carlisle, F. (2006). Marginalisation and ideas of community among Latin American migrants to the UK. *Gender and Development, 14*(2), 235–245.

Carpenter, S. R., Mooney, H. A., Agard, J., Capistrano, D., DeFries, R. S., Díaz, S., & Whyte, A. (2009). Science for managing ecosystem services: Beyond the millennium ecosystem assessment. *Proceedings of the National Academy of Sciences, 106*(5), 1305–1312. https://doi.org/10.1073/pnas.0808772106

Croucher, S. M., Nguyen, T., & Rahmani, D. (2020). Prejudice toward Asian Americans in the Covid-19 pandemic: The effects of social media use in the United States. Frontiers. *Communication, 5*(39). https://doi.org/10.3389/fcomm.2020.00039

Dempster, H., & Zimmer, C. (2020). *Migrant workers in the tourism industry: How has Covid-19 affected them, and what does the future hold? CGD Policy Paper 172.* Center for Global Development.

Dluzewska, A. (2016). Well-being – conceptual background and research practices. *GOD, 25*(4), 547–567.

Fisher, M. (2019). A theory of public well-being. *BMC Public Health, 19*(1), 1–12. https://doi.org/10.1186/s12889-019-7626-z

Garbaye, R. (2005). *Getting into local power: The politics of ethnic minorities in British and French cities* (Vol. 23). Wiley.

Geddes, A., & Scholten, P. (2016). *The politics of migration and immigration in Europe.* Sage.

Gfroerer, J. C., & Tan, L. L. (2003). Substance use among foreign-born youths in the United States: Does the length of residence matter? *American Journal of Public Health, 93*, 1892–1896.

Hargreaves, S. (2020). Europe's migrant containment policies threaten the response to Covid-19. *BMJ, 368*, m1213. https://doi.org/10.1136/bmj.m1213

Hargreaves, S., & Burnett, A. (2008). UK court decision: Healthcare and immigration. *Lancet, 371*, 1823–1824.

Hayward, S. E., Deal, A., Cheng, C., Crawshaw, A., Orcutt, M., Vandrevala, T. F., Norredam, M., Carballo, M., Ciftci, Y., Requena-Méndez, A., Greenaway, C., Carter, J., Knights, F., Mehrotra, A., Seedat, F., Bozorgmehr, K., Veizis, A., Campos-Matos, I., Wurie, F., McKee, M., Kumar, B., Hargreaves, S., & ESCMID Study Group for Infections in Travellers and Migrants (ESGITM). (2021). Clinical outcomes and risk factors for Covid-19 among migrant populations in high-income countries: A systematic review. *Journal of Migration and Health, 3*, 100041. https://doi.org/10.1016/j.jmh.2021.100041

Hobfoll, S. E. (1989). Conservation of resources: A new attempt at conceptualizing stress. *American Psychologist, 44*(3), 513–524. https://doi.org/10.1037/0003-066X.44.3.513

Huo, Y. (2020). Prejudice and discrimination. In J. Jetten, S. D. Reicher, S. A. Haslam, & T. Cruwys (Eds.), *Together apart: The psychology of Covid-19* (pp. 113–118). Sage.

Isaacs, A., Burns, N., Macdonald, S., & O'Donnell, C. A. (2022). 'I don't think there's anything I can do which can keep me healthy': How the UK immigration and asylum system shapes the health & well-being of refugees and asylum seekers in Scotland. *Critical Public Health, 32*(3), 422–432. https://doi.org/10.1080/09581596.2020.1853058

Laverack, G. (2018). The challenge of promoting the health of refugees and migrants in Europe: A review of the literature and urgent policy options. *Challenges, 9*(2), 32. https://doi.org/10.3390/challe9020032

Mangrio E, Carlson E, Zdravkovic S: Understanding experiences of the Swedish health care system from the perspective of newly arrived refugees. BMC Research Notes, 2018 Aug 24: 11:616; doi.org/10.1186/s13104-018-3728-4

Médecins du Monde (European Observatory on Access to Healthcare). (2009). *Access to healthcare for undocumented migrants in 11 European countries: 2008 survey report.* Médecins du Monde.

Médecins Sans Frontières (MSF). (2005). *Experiences of Gomda in Sweden: Exclusion from healthcare for immigrants living without legal status: Results from a survey by Médecins Sans Frotnières.* MSF.

Meleady, R., Hodson, G., & Earle, M. (2021). Person and situation effects in predicting outgroup prejudice and avoidance during the Covid-19 pandemic. *Personality and Individual Differences, 172*, 110593. https://doi.org/10.1016/j.paid.2020.110593

Muoka, M., & Hussier, M. L. (2020). The impact of precarious employment on the health and well-being of UK immigrants: A systematic review. *Journal of Poverty and Social Justice, 28*(3), 337–360.

Myfanwy, M., & Davies, M. (2001). The maternity information concerns of Somali women in the United Kingdom. *Journal of Advanced Nursing, 36*, 237–245.

Nezafat Maldonado, B. M., Collins, J., Blundell, H. J., & Singh, L. (2020). Engaging the vulnerable: A rapid review of public health communication aimed at migrants during the Covid-19 pandemic in Europe. *Journal of Migration and Health, 1–2*, 100004.

Nooria, T., Hargreaves, S., Greenaway, C., Mariekevan, M., der Werfa, R., Driedgere, R., Morton, L., Hui, C., Requena-Mendezh, A., Agbataij, E., Myran, D. T., Pareek, M., Campos-Matos, I., Thoft Nielsen, R., Semenza, J., Nellums, L. B., & Pottie, K. (2021). Strengthening screening for infectious diseases and vaccination among migrants in Europe: What is needed to close the implementation gaps? *Travel Medicine and Infectious Disease, 39*(1), 101715.

Norredam, M., Mygind, A., & Krasnik, A. (2006). Access to health care for asylum seekers in the European Union: A comparative study of country policies. *European Journal of Public Health, 16*(3), 286–290. https://doi.org/10.1093/eurpub/cki191. Epub 2005 Oct 17.

OECD. (2017). Migrants' well-being: Moving to a better life? In *How's life? 2017: Measuring well-being*. OECD. https://doi.org/10.1787/how_life-2017-7-en

OHCHR. (2002/2020). The right of everyone to the enjoyment of the highest attainable standard of physical and mental health Commission on Human Rights: Report on the 58th session, 18 March-26 April 2002. E/2002/23-E/CN.4/2002/200. 2002. pp. 144–147. ESCOR, 2002, Suppl. 3. https://digitallibrary.un.org/record/464198?ln=fr

Papadopoulos, I., Lees, S., Lay, M., & Gebrehiwot, A. (2004). Ethiopian refugees in the UK: Migration, adaptation and settlement experiences and their relevance to health. *Ethnicity and Health, 9*, 55–73.

Parrado, E., Flippen, C., & Uribe, I. (2010). Concentrated disadvantages: Neighbourhood context as a structural risk for Latino immigrants in the USA. In F. Thomas, M. Haour-Knipe, & P. Aggleton (Eds.), *Mobility, sexuality and AIDS* (pp. 40–54). Routledge.

Peiro, M., & Benedict, R. (2010). Migrant health policy, the Portuguese and Spanish EU presidencies. *Eurohealth, 16*(1), 1–4.

Potter, J. L., Burman, M., Tweed, C. D., Vaghela, D., Kunst, H., & Swinglehurst, D. (2020). The NHS visitor and migrant cost recovery programme – A threat to health? *BMC Public Health, 20*(1), 407.

Priebe, S., Sandhu, S., Dias, A., Gaddini, T., Greacen, E., Ioannidis, U., Kluge, A., Krasnik, M., Lamkadem, V., Lorant, R., Riera, P., Savary, A., Soares, M., Stankunas, C., Strassmayr, K. W., Welbel, M., & Bogie, M. (2011). *Good practice in healthcare for migrants: Views and experiences of care professionals in 16 European countries*. BMC Public Health.

Scheppers, E., van Dongen, E., Dekker, J., Geertzen, J., & Dekker, J. (2006). Potential barriers to the use of health services among ethnic minorities: A review. *Family Practice, 23*(3), 325–348.

Sveriges, R., & Lag. (2013:407). om hälso- och sjukvård till vissa utlänningar som vistas i Sverige utan nödvändiga tillstånd. https://www.riksdagen.se/sv/dokument-lagar/dokument/svensk-forfattningssamling/lag-2013407-om-halso%2D%2Doch-sjukvard-till-vissa_sfs-2013-407. Accessed 13 Sep 2022

Trumer, U., Novak-Zezula, S., Metzler, B., & Handler, A. (2010). *Access to health care for undocumented migrants in the EU: A first landscape of now Hereland*. Center for Health and Migration at the Danube University Krems.

UK Government. (2020). *Asylum support*. https://www.gov.uk/asylum-support/what-youll-get.

Van Bavel, J. J., Boggio, P., Capraro, V., Cichocka, A., Cikara, M., Crockett, M., & Willer, R. (2020). Using social and behavioural science to support COVID-19 pandemic response. *PsyArXiv, 4*(5), 460–471. https://doi.org/10.31234/osf.io/y38m9

Wångdahl, J., Lytsy, P., Mårtensson, L., et al. (2014). Health literacy among refugees in Sweden – A cross-sectional study. *BMC Public Health, 14*, 1030. https://doi.org/10.1186/1471-2458-14-1030

WHO/IOM (World Health Organisation and International Organisation for Migration) (2010, March 3). *Health of migrants: The way forward: Report of a global consultation, Madrid.* www.who.int/hae/events/consultation_report_heath_migrants_colour_web.pdf

Louise Dalingwater is a full professor of British politics at Sorbonne Université. Her current research focuses on health policy, healthcare delivery, and well-being in the United Kingdom, with some comparative research on European health systems (notably France) and global health policy research. Recent publications include a book on the UK service economy, a monograph on the NHS, and several book chapters and articles on well-being and health. She has co-edited two publications on well-being: *Well-being: Challenging the Anglo-Saxon Hegemony* (Presses Sorbonne Nouvelle, 2017) and *Well-being: Political Discourse and Policy in the Anglosphere* (Papers in Political Economy, 2019). She is part of the Precision Health Network (an international research project led by the Universities of Lund and Malmo in Sweden). She is also a Chair of the Health Wellness and Society Research Network based in Illinois, United States.

Elisabeth Mangrio is an associate professor at Malmö University. She completed her Ph.D. in Public Health and Social Medicine at Lund University in 2011. She has worked extensively within the research field of migration and health. She is a project manager for the research project *Grow Safely* that investigates the impact of an extended home-visit programme for first-time parents in socially deprived areas in south Sweden. She has done her post-doc within the Support Platform for Migration and Health (MILSA) during 2016–2019 and is a researcher within Precision Health and Everyday Democracy (PHED).

Michael Strange is an associate professor at the Department of Global Political Studies (GPS) at Malmö University. He completed his Ph.D. at the Department of Government at the University of Essex in UK and has a master with Distinction in International Relations. Since 2018, he has directed the STINT-funded international project *Precision Health and Everyday Democracy* (PHED). He has received several major grants within the field of democracy, including focused on healthcare, collaboration, and everyday actors, and is coordinating several research platforms at Malmö University (*REDEM—Rethinking Democracy*; and, *CFM—Collaborative Future-Making*). His published research is highly transdisciplinary, covering both the politics around marginalized migrants, participatory forms of public policy-making, the role of healthcare in relation to democracy, civil society, as well as multi-level policy-making.

Slobodan Zdravkovic is an associate professor in Public Health (epidemiology) at Malmö University. He completed his Ph.D. in epidemiology at the Karolinska Institute in Stockholm, Sweden, in 2006. In his research, he has focused extensively on migration and health and has been a research coordinator of several research projects within the Support Platform for Migration and Health (MILSA).

Chapter 11
Afterword: Tackling Inequalities After the Covid Crisis

Louise Dalingwater

The chapters in this volume suggest how we might tackle the fractures which Covid has created in Europe. Schrecker's chapter paints a stark picture for the future, showing how the pandemic has intensified both economic and health inequalities. In the field of education, Pyżalski and Walter contend that the most important thing is to give specific attention to young people who have to deal with the negative effects of distance education. The most vulnerable require full support with full mental health programmes. The teachers and instructors also need support and guidance because they continue to play an essential role in dealing with the after effects of the health crisis on young people. For Costantini, the virtual experience has not been completely negative for higher education. It is just a question of achieving the right balance between physical and virtual interaction in the future and dealing with specific inequalities, mainly economic ones, for both students and academics at the start of their careers. Verdiyeva et al.'s study of children with severe disabilities shows that ongoing support for parents who have had to take over the role of educator is important. In Lestrade's analysis of the workplace, a more flexible approach, which allows employees to work from home, should be continued even though this still excludes certain segments of the population who do not have the opportunity to work from home. Lazarashvili et al. and Boullet and Guillaumond's chapters contend that continued intervention from the government is necessary to alleviate the negative and unequal effects of the economic downturn on the population. The state's role in ensuring the well-being and welfare of the population is essential. As regards health interventions, Lillo-Crespo underlines how important it is to ensure that response systems are in place well before emergencies strike to enable organized and coordinated action which can in effect benefit the most vulnerable in society. Dalingwater et al. reiterate this in their chapter by arguing

L. Dalingwater (✉)
Sorbonne Université, Paris, France
e-mail: louise.dalingwater@sorbonne-universite.fr

that there is a need to ensure that the lessons of Covid-19, during which inequities and weaknesses in healthcare have been exposed, continue to be dealt with to ensure that we become resilient to future pandemics.

The Covid-19 epidemic has increased calls for inclusive development given that the response strategies have been in many ways an "every man for himself" approach and a lack of solidarity with poorer nations but also poorer people in rich nations (Gupta et al., 2021). Inclusive development is the process of including marginalized people, sectors, and countries into social political and economic processes in order to enhance human well-being, social and environmental sustainability and empowerment (Gupta et al., 2021, p. 543). Ultimately it is a wider agenda approach than the current well-being agenda. Multi-sectoral and community engagement is necessary to reduce inequities and marginalization. Only through a multi-sectoral engagement can risk to infection and long-term poor health be dealt with (WHO, 2020). The WHO calls for an engagement from national and local government, the media, employers, the private sector, and the third sector (NGOs, civil society ...) (WHO, 2020).

The question is whether global governance systems will be redesigned or continue to work according to pre-crisis systems of governance. The danger of continuing with previous frameworks is that they have proved to be inefficient in dealing with major health crises. As Gupta et al. (2021) underline, the International Agenda 2030 and the Sustainable Development Goals (SDGs) which aim to accelerate progress in fighting communicable diseases and epidemics and ensure access to essential medicines and vaccines do not have sufficiently wide frames to address the issues of inclusive health relating to social, ecological, and relational issues.

One of the main recommendations of the recent Marmot report was to increase public health funding significantly and move towards a public health system that focuses more widely on improving living and working conditions (Marmot et al., 2020). Taking a rights-based approach, Gupta and Lebel (2010, 2020) call for a socially inclusiveness approach to ensure that all people have access to public goods and services which cover their basic needs in terms of food, water, energy, health, education, income, and work. This should also include the fair allocation of resources among different socio-economic categories, across countries and generations. Rather than just focusing on who is vulnerable and responding on an *ad hoc* basis to the needs of these populations, Gupta and Lebel (2020) underline the importance of studying the drivers which have caused this vulnerability and the unequal division of resources.

Rashid and Pepperelli go much further and argue a case for implementing a full-scale degrowth plan. They claim that the scale of destruction which has ensued from this pandemic was not inevitable. The pandemic has exposed weaknesses in social, health, and economic systems in the global north. Deprived populations have experienced poorer health outcomes. A solution to rising inequalities can only come from a transition to an alternative economic system. The current one has endangered lives and widened inequalities. The pandemic has indeed led to a renewal of support for basic income and wealth taxes, financing a transition to a more equitable economy through taxes on capital, inheritance, financial transactions, and polluting activities. Added to this is a call for degrowth, a reduction of economic activities, and an increase in economic support structures. This theory calls into question the idea that increasing growth through a focus on GDP can lead to improved well-being for populations. GDP is considered to be a flawed indicator because as Bobby Kennedy underlined in a speech as early as 1968:

> Gross national product does not allow for the health of our children, the quality of their education or the joy of their play. It does not include the beauty of our poetry or the strength of our marriages, the intelligence of our public debate or the integrity of our public officials. It measures neither our wit nor our courage, neither our wisdom nor our learning, neither our compassion nor our devotion to our country, it measures everything in short, except that which makes life worthwhile (Kennedy, 1968).

Both degrowth and well-being theorists contend that we need to go beyond the emphasis on GDP as a benchmark for the well-being of society in line with Kennedy's observation. Yet the well-being theories that have been developed more recently which underline that GDP is an inadequate measure of wealth, have led to a promotion of subjective and individual well-being rather than developing policies to tackle inequalities. Degrowth theories debunk the idea that GDP growth leads to a trickle down of wealth and a closing of the gap between the rich and poor. They also provide collective solutions to tackle inequalities head on. They call for greater preventative measures for illness through a wider community health approach.

In addition to degrowth proposals, there are also calls to reconstruct the social and economic systems through "build back better" projects. Proponents argue that there is a temptation, as we emerge from the crisis, to defend neoliberal economic systems and ideologies and encourage a reboot of growth and a reduction in market regulations, or even the implementation of austerity measures to reduce public debt. However, the risk is that this will further exacerbate inequalities in economic, health, and educational performances. The "build back better" approach is therefore the idea that we should see the crisis as an opportunity to transform our economic and social structures. In order to achieve effective and collective well-being, its proponents argue we need to remain within planetary boundaries to achieve satisfaction for all including the most vulnerable in our society (Raworth, 2017). New institutions should be created to support collective well-being and ecological sustainability. Yet, in this volume, Schrecker voices our underlying fear that while the rhetoric of "building back better" is well intentioned, initiatives to reduce inequalities may well be doomed to fail especially given present and future environmental challenges.

References

Gupta, J., & Lebel, L. (2010). Access and allocation in earth system governance: Water and climate change compared. *International Environmental Agreements: Politics, Law and Economics, 10*, 377–395. https://doi.org/10.1007/s10784-010-9139-1

Gupta, J., & Lebel, L. (2020). Access and allocation in earth system governance: Justice, inclusive development and the sustainable development goals. *International Environmental Agreements: Politics, Law and Economics, 20*, 393–410. https://doi.org/10.1007/s10784-010-9139-1

Gupta, J., Bavinck, M., Ros-Tonen, M., Asubonteng, K., Bosch, H., van Ewijk, E., Hordijk, M., Van Leynseele, Y., Lopes Cardozo, M., Miedema, E., Pouw, N., Rammelt, C., Scholtens, J., Vegelin, C., & Verrest, H. (2021). Covid-19, poverty and inclusive development. *World Development, 145*, 105527. https://doi.org/10.1016/j.worlddev.2021.105527

Kennedy, B. (1968). *MR 89–34. Miscellaneous Recordings*, John F. Kennedy Presidential Library.

Marmot, M., Allen, J., Boyce, T., Goldblatt, P., & Morrison, J. (2020). *Health equity in England: The marmot review 10 years on*. Institute of Health Equity.

Raworth, K. (2017). A doughnut for the anthropocene: Humanity's compass in the 21st century. *The Lancet Planetary Health, 1*(2), e48–e49. https://doi.org/10.1016/S2542-5196(17)30028-1

World Health Organization. (2020). *Malnutrition (2020)*. https://www.who.int/news-room/fact-sheets/detail/malnutrition 2020.

Louise Dalingwater is a full professor of British politics at Sorbonne Université. Her current research focuses on health policy, healthcare delivery and well-being in the United Kingdom, with some comparative research on European health systems (notably France) and global health policy research. Recent publications include a book on the UK service economy, a monograph on the NHS, and several book chapters and articles on well-being and health. She has coedited two publications on well-being: *Well-being: Challenging the Anglo-Saxon Hegemony* (Presses Sorbonne Nouvelle, 2017) and *Well-being: Political Discourse and Policy in the Anglosphere* (Papers in Political Economy, 2019). She is part of the Precision Health Network (an international research project led by the Universities of Lund and Malmo in Sweden). She is also Chair of the Health Wellness and Society Research Network based in Illinois, United States.

The manufacturer's authorised representative in the EU is Springer
Nature Customer Service Centre GmbH, Europaplatz 3, 69115 Heidelberg,
Germany. If you have any concerns regarding our products, please
contact ProductSafety@springernature.com

Printed and bound by CPI Group (UK) Ltd, Croydon, CR0 4YY

29/04/2026

02099522-0001